OPTIMAL GUIDE TO YOUR BEST PHYSIQUE:

RAW TRUTH BEHIND NUTRITION & TRAINING

KAMERON GEORGE

Photo Credits: Veronchick84/ Alexey lysenko/ Design36/ Dedek R.Iegosyn/ Andrey Makurin/ Joshua Resnick/ Stas Tolstnev/ Velirina/ Slonme/ Mikhail Grachikov/ Aliaksei smalenski/ Lightspring/ Dm7/ Spaxiax/ Ambient Ideas/ Spaxiax/ Peogeo/ Sergio Stakhnyk/ Mopic/ Picsfive/Aaron Amat/ Maraze/ Brent Hofacker/ Sarsmis/Shutterstock.com

To my H.S. track coach Mac—

*Without your motivation and belief,
my success would not be possible.*

TABLE OF CONTENTS

I. OPTIMAL NUTRITION

II. OPTIMAL TRAINING

III. OPTIMAL FITNESS THEORY

ABOUT THE AUTHOR

Born and raised in Brooklyn, New York, I grew up playing basketball, baseball, soccer, track & field and cross-country. As a rookie track runner in the 11th grade, I became a New York City Public School Champion in the 1-mile, 2-mile, 4x800 and cross-country races throughout my last two years of high school. These accomplishments led to athletic and academic scholarships to Norfolk State University where I obtained bachelor degrees in electronic engineering and mathematics. During the summers of college and in between seasons of track and cross-country, I followed a home workout program in hopes of returning to campus with an amazing physique. I was able to attain decent results but it wasn't what I imagined it to be. I began to persistently search the web for new information on nutrition and training in hopes of finding a shortcut to a great physique. I often discovered something that I can improve on, which led to occasional changes to my routine. In attempt to see faster results, I would just run harder and train my abs more frequently.

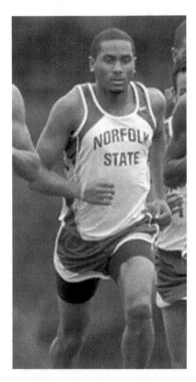

Hundreds of miles and many ab workouts later, I was still left with skinny arms and barely visible abs hiding under a rounded stomach. I was aggravated knowing that I put in the hard work and patience that every successful athlete preaches about, yet I was unable to transform my "skinny-fat" physique. After figuring out that nutrition played a huge part in achieving my dream physique, I began tracking calories. Though I easily lost weight, I faced issues such as muscle loss, frequent food-binges, crankiness, and a slightly more defined version of my same physique but still not what I imagined. Determined to reach my goal, this led to years of continuous research on anything fitness related. With many trials and errors, I eventually discovered where I went wrong and was able to shape my physique into what I was always wanted it to be. In this book, I share the valuable information that will lead you straight to the physique you want without the time-wasting issues I had to go through. I've grown to thoroughly enjoy the science behind how the human body works and implementing research to efficiently improve my health and physique. My passion is now fulfilled as a personal online fitness coach where I am able to help others achieve their fitness goals.

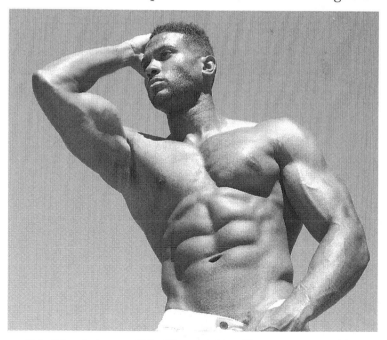

"Nothing is impossible. The word itself says I'm possible"
~ **Audrey Hepburn**

PURPOSE OF THE BOOK

This straight-to-the-point book revolves around working smart to attain the results you really want. If people would learn more about how their body functions towards their goals, they would save a lot of unnecessary time and effort. These guided tips and advice serve those who have the motivation to work hard in order to acquire their goal physique and are looking for the most *optimal* way to accomplish their goal. People who will find this book extremely beneficial include those who don't like to "beat around the bush", are interested in the best of quality, or who have attempted to reach their fitness goal several times but have yet to see significant results. For these readers, this guide will allow them to throw any excuses out of the window and take control of achieving their goal physique.

The purpose of this book is to provide quality comprehensive information on how to burn fat and/or build muscle while staying healthy. Nutrition has a major role in this book since working out while paying no attention to how you eat will take you down a road of little to no results. My duty is to show people that they do not have to be limited to certain foods while trying to reach their goal. *Optimal Guide To Your Best Physique* exploits the common habits that are unnecessary, while explaining the ones that actually matter towards achieving the physique you aspire. This information will save a tremendous amount of time towards any fitness goal for beginners or anyone who already has training experience and would like to advance their knowledge on nutrition and training. The basic titles of each section and informative points are structured in a way that the reader can easily comprehend. Think of this guide as a blueprint and vital resource to acquiring your desired physique. With this book, any confusion about reaching your goal is cleared up and the only thing left to do is the work itself.

"Believe you can, and you're halfway there" ~ **Theodore Roosevelt**

Optimal - the best, most favorable, or desirable, especially under some restriction

With many ways to pursue your goal, there is always a better or smarter way to get the job done. The role of this guide is intended to produce *optimal* results in terms of nutrition and training. This information will help you filter through the common buzz among the fitness community and fully understand the basics of how the body is able to burn fat and build muscle. This is a simple guide to reaching your fitness goal in the quickest and most efficient way. With the knowledge presented, you'd be sure to take on your goal with total awareness and complete confidence.

I. OPTIMAL NUTRITION

*"A journey of a thousand miles,
begins with a single step"* ~ **Lao Tzo**

EATING HEALTHY VS. ACHIEVING YOUR GOAL PHYSIQUE

With the thought of achieving a great physique, people instantly think of eating healthy. Yet eating healthy foods doesn't necessarily mean you're achieving your goal physique. While acquiring your best physique doesn't exactly mean you're eating healthy. To eat healthy generally means you provide your body with enough nutrients to function efficiently. Your body demands a specific amount of micronutrients (vitamins and minerals) and macronutrients (fats, proteins, and carbs) in order to work at its best ability. It is your responsibility to fulfill your body's nutritional requirements in order to maintain good health. Achieving a great physique usually involves losing fat or gaining muscle. In order to lose fat, an individual must be in a calorie deficit where your body burns more calories than the amount of calories you eat and drink. Gaining weight requires one to do the opposite, where in a calorie surplus you consume more calories than the amount your body burns.

Although eating healthy foods has endless benefits, it is just as important to fulfill the requirement of achieving your fitness goal. For example, if your goal is to burn fat and you eat 10,000 calories worth of vegetables each day, you're eating healthy but are consuming too many calories to accomplish your goal. Therefore, it is ideal to eat towards your goal physique while maintaining good health. Both of these objectives are done by consuming the amount of calories that will allow you to accomplish your fitness goal while acquiring sufficient micronutrients and macronutrients so your body can function efficiently.

WHAT IS A CALORIE?

You hear about calories all the time, but exactly what does it mean? A calorie is a unit that measures energy. The food you eat isn't measured in weight or size, but by how much energy it contains. When you hear something contains 100 calories, it's a way of describing how much energy your body could get from eating or drinking it[1]. Just as the amount of gas pumped into a car is measured in gallons, the different food or drinks you consume is measured in calories. The body breaks down food in a unique way, so the amount of calories is a way of knowing how much energy your body will get from anything you eat or drink. 'Calorie' is simply a technical word for 'energy'.

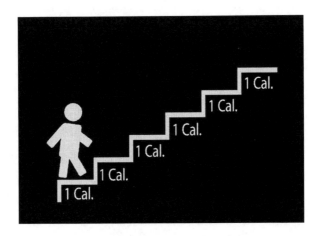

ARE CALORIES BAD FOR YOU?

Calories are not bad for you since your body needs them for energy. Yet eating too many calories and not burning enough of them off through physical activity can lead to weight gain over time. Consuming too little calories over time will not allow your body to function properly and can negatively affect your health. Foods such as lettuce contain very few calories (1 cup of shredded lettuce has less than 10 calories), while foods like peanuts contain a lot of calories (½ cup of peanuts has 427 calories) [1]. Knowing how many calories your body needs each day will help you choose which foods are best for you.

HOW DOES YOUR BODY USE CALORIES?

Your body needs calories just to stay alive and operate properly. This energy is used for basic functions such as keeping your heart beating and lungs breathing. Calories are essential for all basic and complex functions including the regulation of body temperature and the operation of every cell in your body. The more activity you do is the more calories you burn. Your body also needs calories in order to grow and develop. You burn calories without even thinking about it such as during the digestion of food, recovery of muscles after exercise, and even while you sleep.

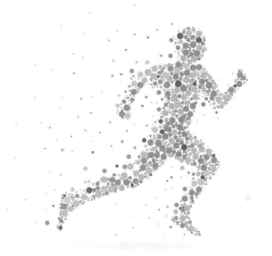

HOW MANY CALORIES DO YOU NEED?

People differ in size and have different metabolisms, so the amount of calories a person should consume will vary depending on several factors. These factors include a person's height, weight, age, and daily activity level. The bigger a person is, the more calories that person may need, vice versa. Even though two people can have the same body measurements, the amount of calories they need can differ because of the way their body metabolizes what they consume. Calorie calculators are available online, which can be used to determine how many calories your body needs based on the necessary factors. If you eat more calories than your body needs, then the extra calories are converted into fat. If you eat less calories then you need, then your body uses your stored body fat as the energy it needs to function. Understanding the amount of calories you need will help you better control your weight.

MACRO BASICS

Macronutrients or macros are **carbohydrates**, **fats**, and **protein**. With the term "macro" meaning very large, these three nutrients are responsible for providing calories (the only other substance that provides calories is alcohol but is not a macronutrient since we do not need it for survival). Anything you eat is broken down to these three macronutrients. Your body does not recognize the food you eat as "chicken, rice, salad, etc". Instead, your body sees whatever you consume as a carb, fat, or protein. This is the reason you find these macronutrients written in bold letters on the nutrition label of any food or drink product.

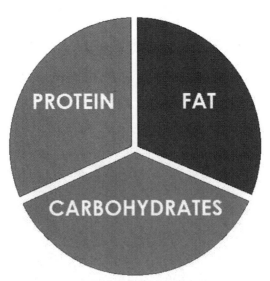

Calories are made up of three macros

WHAT IS A CARB?

A carbohydrate is your body's primary source of energy. There are two types of carbs, simple and complex. A simple carb supplies your body with quick energy, but doesn't last long. A complex carb takes longer to break down in your body, yet is a long-lasting source of energy. Neither simple nor complex carb is bad for you. They can both be used to your advantage throughout the day. Upon waking up in the morning, chances are you haven't had anything to eat for the last few hours you've been asleep. Therefore it can be a good idea to consume simple carbs for the immediate energy. If you plan on being out of the house for a few hours, complex carbs would be a good choice for its long-lasting steady energy. So incorporating both types of carbs in your diet can allow you to better control your levels of energy throughout the day.

Examples of complex carbs include whole grains such as whole wheat bread, oatmeal, and brown rice along with other foods such as sweet potato and beans. Simple carbs include foods such as fruits, white bread, white rice, white potatoes, vegetables, juice, pop tarts, etc. Sugar is a simple carbohydrate that comes in different forms such as glucose, fructose, lactose, sucrose, etc. Although both simple and complex carbs are eventually broken down to sugar in the body, digestion and absorption are the main differences between the two types.

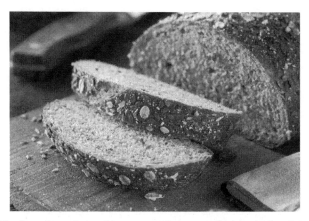

Whole wheat bread is a popular complex carbohydrate

WHAT IS PROTEIN?

Protein helps build and repair tissue while playing a role in various cell functions in the body. It is a major component for growing hair, nails, muscle and other parts of the body. Amino acids are the building blocks of protein. A complete protein consists of all 20 amino acids, while the absence of one or more amino acid is considered an incomplete protein. Complete proteins are mainly found in meats such as chicken, beef, steak, fish as well as eggs, milk, and whey protein. Foods such as grains, nuts, seeds, or legumes are considered incomplete proteins. It is recommended to consume at least 0.8 - 1.2 grams of protein per 1 pound of your bodyweight for optimal muscle growth. With many different types of protein on the market ranging from the source, absorption rate, and process of filtration, any complete protein is beneficial for the growth and repair of muscle. Poultry, fish, dairy, legume, soy, whey and other sources of proteins have their differences but any complete protein is of great benefit for building and repairing muscle. The key is to get enough protein to fulfill your body's requirement for optimal growth.

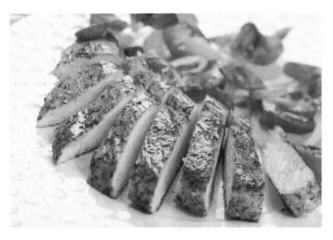

Chicken breast is one of many complete proteins

WHAT IS FAT?

Fat controls hormones, aides in the transport of cells, and makes it possible for other nutrients to complete tasks in the body. Fat is also your body's secondary source of energy. When your body doesn't have enough carbs readily available, it uses fat as another source of fuel. Therefore, the idea of burning fat is to limit the amount of primary energy (carbs) so the body can use its secondary source for energy (body fat). Different types of fats include saturated, polyunsaturated, monounsaturated, and trans-fat. It is recommended to stay away from trans-fat due to its health disadvantages. While each type of fat has its pros and cons, it is useful to pay attention to the total amount of fat in a product. Foods that contain a high amount of fat include butter, peanut butter, oils, avocado, and nuts. Consuming low amounts of fat over time can cause hormone levels to become unbalanced, making it important to get enough even while trying to burn fat. The amount of fat needed daily can vary anywhere from 15% to over 40% of total calories depending on the individual and fitness goal.

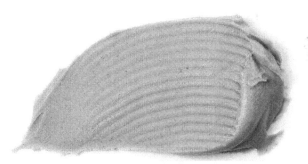

Peanut butter contains a high amount of fat

WHY TRACK MACROS?

QUALITY OF WEIGHT LOSS OR WEIGHT GAIN

If you are in a calorie deficit where your body burns more calories than you consume, then you will lose weight. This does not necessarily ensure that all the weight you lose will only come from fat. Your body is made up of lean mass, fat, and water. This means any weight that is lost or gained can come from any of these three. When dropping weight you risk losing muscle, and when gaining weight you risk putting on excessive fat. Not tracking macros puts you at a higher risk for muscle loss and fat gain because you wouldn't know how many calories you are getting. Consuming the right amount of fat, protein, and carbs will help to ensure that you maintain muscle while losing fat, and limit the increase of body fat when adding muscle.

MORE ENERGY, BETTER MOOD

Carbohydrates are the body's main source of energy, so having too little carbs over time can leave you feeling tired and lead to poor workout performance. By properly setting up your macros, you maximize the amount of carbs you are able to consume while efficiently burning fat. If you can eat more food while losing fat, then why not take advantage. Fat is responsible for controlling your hormones, so not having enough may cause an imbalance which can lead to mood swings and other unwanted symptoms. It is common to fall short of your daily fat requirements by only eating "clean" foods which typically contain little to no fat. Consuming insufficient fat and/or carbs over time can cause you to feel extremely miserable. To think losing weight is already a challenge, why make it harder on yourself to reach your goal.

MACROS ARE LIKE MONEY

Would you rather someone tell you how to spend your money or would you want to spend it the way you want to. You should feel free to buy expensive things as long as you remain within your budget. Your macros are like your daily budget and you can spend it any way you like. By staying within your daily macronutrient requirement, you have the freedom to eat the foods you enjoy without interrupting the progress of your fitness goal. This method may be more sustainable to a normal lifestyle than following a meal plan that is known to limit your food choices. If you happen to travel somewhere that doesn't have the foods available in your meal plan you may be confused on what you should to eat. Yet someone knowing how many macronutrients they're allowed will be more flexible to eat different foods in any situation. Any proper meal plan should be structured using a customized set of macronutrients, and then created with specific foods. Why not use the same customized macros and fill them with an unlimited range of foods that you love to eat.

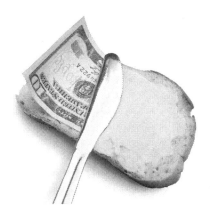

NO TIME WASTED

Another major reason why it's important to keep track of your macronutrients is to make sure you are not moving too fast or too slow towards your fitness goal. Losing weight too fast can result in muscle loss and low energy, while moving too slow can prolong seeing results in your physique. By tracking your macronutrient intake, you are able to know exactly how much to consume so your weight changes at your desired pace. It is a greater benefit to know your macronutrient intake if your fitness goal has a deadline since it helps ensure that you meet your goal in time. In other words, you are nearly in full control of transforming your physique at the pace you want. Tracking macros is proven to be more effective than the "eating clean" method when attempting to burn fat. What if you are eating "clean" and your weight loss eventually plateaus? Do you just eat "cleaner"? Keeping track of your macronutrients offers more control over your bodyweight and allows you to make accurate adjustments so you can maintain progression towards your goal with little to no time wasted.

FOOD AWARENESS

Understanding macros makes you more aware of your choices in food. Knowing the amount of macronutrients in the food you eat is not only beneficial for short-term progress but for a lifetime. You will be eating food for the rest of your life. Therefore, understanding the amount of calories in the foods you eat will allow you better control over the outcome of your physique. Once you're able to see your daily intake of calories in comparison to how much your body needs, you will have a better understanding of why your physique looks the way it is. By knowing the amount of calories your body is allowed, you can know how much food will cause a change in your physique rather than guessing.

EASIER THAN YOU THINK

Although accurately tracking your macros each day is ideal, you don't have to be perfect in order to see significant progress towards your goal. The macronutrient goals for an individual is a calculated estimate of how much you should consume in order to stay on pace towards your goal. If you miss your macros by a few grams a couple days out of the week, you can still see good results. Instead of losing 2 pounds of fat for the week, you might just lose 1.9 pounds of fat. It's not perfect, but that's still great progress towards your goal. An individual can often mentally track their macros if they already know the amounts in the food they frequently eat. Tracking macros can also be viewed as a daily puzzle of food. It can actually be fun fitting the different foods you enjoy into your daily macronutrient goals.

OPTIMAL

You can still achieve a great physique without tracking your macros, but it is more like hopeful guessing that can produce sub-*optimal* results. Tracking macros makes the difference between hoping and ensuring that you achieve your goal in the most efficient and accurate way. The idea is to control the right balance of nutrients so you can maintain healthy progression towards your fitness goal. From the aspects of time, stress, and quality of results, tracking macros is proven to be the most *optimal* way to better your physique.

"What you do today can improve all your tomorrows"
~ Ralph Marston

WHEN TO EAT CARBS?

If carbs provide energy and you use energy in every aspect of your daily life, then knowing which foods are carbs and when to eat them is worth taking a little time to learn. Understanding the power of carbs allows you to take full control of your energy levels and make smarter food choices throughout the day. One of the most beneficial times to consume carbs is in the morning. This is mainly because chances are you've been sleeping for the past few hours and haven't had anything to eat. Therefore, it is ideal to consume simple carbs for the immediate energy as well as complex carbs for long-lasting energy. Another beneficial time to consume carbs is before and after working out. Consuming carbs pre-workout will support your training performance while having carbs post-workout allows for *optimal* muscle recovery and stabilization of blood-sugar levels. It is fine to eat carbs at any other time, but these are the main points of the day that are most beneficial.

You may have heard of the theory that eating carbs at night is going to cause you to gain fat because your body won't process the food while you sleep. Though this misconception has been proven false, it can be a good strategy to consume most of your carbs when you need them the most, which is usually during the day. Although most people are usually less active at night, it is okay to eat carbs as long as you meet your required amount for the day.

WHEN TO EAT PROTEIN?

Consumption of protein should ideally be spread throughout the day. There is no specific limit to the amount of protein an individual should eat in one serving. There have been several studies showing that consuming protein in large portions compared to small portions were found to produce the same results in both muscle growth and weight loss as long as the daily protein requirement is met. In other words, the amount of protein you consume in one sitting is insignificant as long as you hit your total protein requirement by the end of the day. The most beneficial times to consume protein are before and after training. The key is to keep amino acids (protein) active in the bloodstream at all times. Overall, it is recommended to divide your daily protein requirement into each of the meals you plan to have for the day. For example, if you know you need 150 grams of protein each day, you can split that amount into 3 meals with 50 grams of protein or have 5 meals with 30 grams of protein.

HOW IS FAT BURNED?

Fat is your body's secondary source of energy. This source is mainly used when your body doesn't have enough carbs available. Therefore, in order to burn the fat stored in your body, you must limit the amount of carbs you consume so that you begin to use fat as energy. This is why being in a caloric deficit where you eat or drink fewer calories than the amount of calories you burn each day, results in your body using its own stored fat for the energy it needs.

One pound of fat is equal to 3,500 calories. So in order to lose 1 pound of fat, you must burn 3,500 calories more than the amount of calories your body needs to maintain its weight. Creating a 3,500 calorie deficit in one day can be extreme for most people, but if you portion this amount over the course of 7 days, it results in a reasonable 500 calorie deficit each day. The key to burning fat is to consistently maintain a caloric deficit over time. If you are able to maintain a caloric deficit of 500 calories each day for 7 days, then you will burn 1 pound of fat. The larger the calorie deficit is, the faster you will lose weight. You can lose 2 pounds of fat in a week by increasing the deficit to 1,000 calories each day.

When thinking of creating a caloric deficit for fat loss, most people initially think of eating fewer calories. Though this method is useful, it is not the only way to create a calorie deficit. An individual can consume the same amount of calories they've already been eating, yet create a calorie deficit by burning calories through exercise. The idea of creating a calorie deficit can be compared to methods of saving money. You can save money by working extra hours to increase your income, or you can simply spend less money. In order to avoid exhausting hours of extra work or drastically cutting how much you spend, it is a good idea to combine both methods and work a little more while spending a little less. A similar method can be applied to burning fat where you can combine exercise and consuming fewer calories in order to efficiently create a calorie deficit.

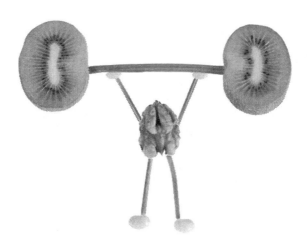

"The only thing standing between you and your goal is the bullsh*t story you keep telling yourself as to why you can't achieve it"
~ Jordan Bellfort

CUT VS. MAINTENANCE VS. BULK

A cut, maintenance, and bulk are different conditional states that control the outcome of your weight based on the amount of calories you consume over time. In other words, you can eat less, more, or equal to the amount of calories your body burns each day in order to adjust the composition of your physique. When you consume the same amount of calories as your body burns each day, you will remain the same weight. This is known as being in a caloric **maintenance** state (*Meal B)*, which most people tend to follow. Your body usually regulates this state by telling you that you're hungry when you consume too little calories, and tells you that you're full when you have had too many calories. No fat loss is generated during this state but moderate muscle growth can occur.

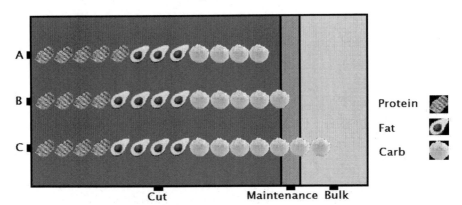

In a **cut** (caloric deficit), you consume less calories than your body needs to maintain its weight. In this state, your body doesn't have enough carbs to supply your body's energy demand causing it to use stored fat for secondary energy. This causes a decrease in body fat, allowing you to look leaner. Though being in this caloric state can tone your physique, the rate of muscle growth is usually at a minimum. The goal of a cut is to lose body fat while maintaining muscle. The best way to ensure that you maintain muscle mass during a cut is to incorporate weight training and consume a sufficient amount of protein. People looking to lose weight or achieve a defined physique should focus on being in a cut (*Meal A)*. In a **bulk** (caloric surplus), you consume more calories than your body needs to maintain its weight. Due to the extra calories provided, your body has more energy to focus on tasks such as muscle recovery. Though you gain muscle quicker, it is common to gain some amount of fat while in a caloric surplus. The goal of a bulk is to gain muscle while adding the least amount of fat. People who are looking to gain weight should focus on being in a bulk (*Meal C*). For beginners at weight training, rapid muscle growth can occur during a bulk, maintenance, or cut granted enough protein is provided and the muscles are properly stimulated.

CLEAN FOODS VS. DIRTY FOODS

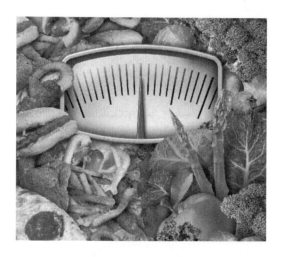

A "clean" food is often described as an unprocessed or whole food that is full of vitamins and minerals, generally containing little to no fat or sugar. A "dirty" food is usually processed, contains little to no micronutrients, and usually high in fat or sugar. Categorizing foods as "dirty" or "clean" is impractical and is more of an informal word used to describe its contents. There are many articles that discuss the top ten good foods and bad foods, but these are the critiques of a specific food without considering the other foods you eat. The problem is that you don't eat foods in isolation; you consume various foods as part of a diet. There is no such thing as a good or bad food, but there is such thing as a good or bad diet. Avoiding individual foods such as bread or dairy for the hopes of burning fat is insignificant if your entire diet doesn't coordinate with your fitness goal. The key is to focus more on the amount of nutrients aligned with your goal rather than choosing between a clean or dirty food. These nutrients include the total carbs, fat, and protein along with the amount of vitamins and minerals in the food you eat.

"Things work best for those who make the best of how things work out"
~ John Wooden

VITAMINS AND MINERALS

Vitamins and minerals make up the micronutrients that help to make every process in your body possible. They strengthen the immune system, support growth, and also help metabolize the food you eat. Vitamins are organic compounds, meaning they can be found in all living things. Minerals are inorganic elements that are derived from soil and water. All vitamins are necessary or required by your body, whereas only some minerals are essential nutrients. Each nutrient is responsible for specific cellular processes that help manage the body's health. By consuming a variety of micronutrients each day, it further ensures that your body will operate efficiently.

Once you've met your body's daily requirement for vitamins and minerals, consuming excess amounts will only be stored in fat or excreted. Vitamins fall into two groups, fat-soluble and water-soluble. Water-soluble vitamins need to dissolve in water before your body can absorb them. Since your body cannot store them, it is important to consume sufficient amounts every day. Fat-soluble vitamins are stored in the body's cells and are not excreted as easily as water-soluble vitamins. They do not need to be consumed as often as water-soluble vitamins, although adequate amounts are needed. If you consume too much of a fat-soluble vitamin, it could become toxic to your body. Many people often fall short of their daily micronutrient intake, so supplementing with a multivitamin serves as insurance in case you haven't met all your vitamin and mineral requirements from food.

16

VITAMINS

Nutrient	Function	Food Sources
Vitamin A	Supports healthy skin, teeth, bones, soft tissue, good vision, and mucous membranes.	Animal sources, milk, cheese, butter, eggs, liver, dark green vegetables, mangos, cantaloupe, carrots, winter squash, sweet potatoes, pumpkin
Vitamin B1 (Thiamine)	Needed to metabolize carbohydrates. Supports function of heart, nervous system, and muscle coordination.	Whole grain cereal, pork, poultry, nuts, beans, seeds, breads, rice, pasta
Vitamin B2 (Riboflavin)	Needed to break down carbs, fats, and protein. Promotes growth of healthy hair, skin, eyes, and nails.	Spinach, yogurt, mushrooms, almonds, eggs, turkey, soybeans, breads, whole-grain cereals
Vitamin B3 (Niacin)	Needed to break down carbs, fats, and protein. Improves cardiovascular, brain, and nervous system health.	Meat, poultry, fish, whole-grain or enriched breads, cereals, mushrooms, asparagus, peanut butter, green peas, avocado
Vitamin B5 (Pantothenic-acid)	Needed to break down carbs, fats, and protein. Supports growth of hormones and immune system.	Whole grains, meats, egg yolk, mushrooms, sweet potato, lentils, broccoli
Vitamin B6 (Pyridoxine)	Aides in breakdown of carbs, fats, and protein. Helps maintain the health of nerves, skin, and red blood cells.	Meat, fish, poultry, vegetables, fruits
Vitamin B7 (Biotin)	Needed to break down carbs, fats, and protein. Supports healthy skin, hair, nails, nerves, and nervous system.	Mushrooms, tuna, turkey, salmon, eggs, cheese, cauliflower, whole grains
Vitamin B9 (Folic acid)	Protects and develops nervous system. Supports production of DNA and new cells.	Leafy green vegetables, legumes, seeds, beets
Vitamin B12 (Cobalamin)	Supports normal brain and nervous system functioning. Helps metabolize DNA synthesis and energy production.	Meat, poultry, fish, seafood, eggs, milk, cheese

Vitamin C	Serves as an antioxidant. Needed for the growth and repair of all tissue. Supports brain and collagen health.	Citrus fruits, strawberries, watermelon, papaya, mangos, broccoli, spinach, green/red peppers, potatoes, and tomatoes
Vitamin D	Helps your body absorb calcium and supports strong, healthy bones	Sunlight, egg yolks, liver, fish oil, dairy products, tuna, sunflower seeds
Vitamin E	Serves as a natural antioxidant. Protects cell walls, keeps red blood cells and nerves healthy.	Almonds, peanuts, sunflower seeds, eggs, spinach, avocado, asparagus, olive oil
Vitamin K	Needed for proper blood clotting.	Kale, asparagus, prune, olive oil, broccoli, cabbage, spinach, fermented dairy

MINERALS

Calcium	Need for bone growth, blood clotting, and muscle contraction.	Milk, dairy products such as yogurt and cheese, kale
Iron	Helps red blood cells transport oxygen to all parts of the body.	Red meat, fish, poultry, beans, flour, grains, raisins, dark leafy vegetables
Magnesium	Helps muscles and nerves function, regulates heart rhythm, and keep bones strong. Also helps create energy and process proteins.	Whole grains, nuts, seed, potatoes, beans avocados, milk, dark leafy vegetables, bananas
Phosphorus	Helps make healthy bones and teeth. Required in every cell membrane of the body to aid in making energy.	Most foods but high in dairy products, meat, fish, nuts, beans.
Potassium	Helps with heart, muscle, and nervous system functions. Aides in the balance of water in blood and body tissue.	Broccoli, dark leafy greens, bananas, potatoes, beans, citrus fruits
Zinc	Needed to support immune system, cell growth, and breakdown of carbohydrates. Also needed for use of senses like smell and taste.	Nuts, seeds, red meat poultry, seafood, whole grains, milk and other dairy products
Chromium	Helps move glucose from the bloodstream and into cells to be used as energy.	Broccoli, green beans, tomatoes, whole grains, potatoes, oranges, meat, poultry, fish, beans, eggs.

Sodium	Helps keep the water and electrolyte balance in the body. Regulates blood pressure and cellular work. Vital to the function of nerves and muscles.	Salt, sauces, salad dressing, pickles, crab, canned vegetables
Copper	Helps absorb iron. Plays role in energy production.	Seafood, nuts, seeds, beans, whole grains
Iodine	Helps make thyroid hormones and maintain cell metabolism.	Seafood, iodized salt, dairy products
Fluorine	Increases bone density, fights infections and reduces incidence of tooth decay.	Asparagus, avocados, carrots, spinach, garlic, nuts, tomatoes, cabbage, dates
Selenium	Antioxidant properties protect cells from damage.	Brazil nuts, seafood, poultry, beef, whole wheat, seeds, mushrooms

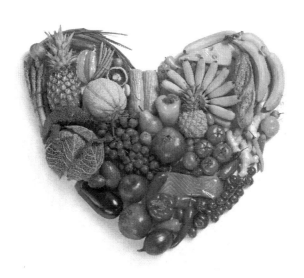

IMPORTANCE OF FIBER

Fiber is the part of plant foods that our bodies can't digest or absorb. There are two kinds of dietary fiber, insoluble and soluble. Soluble fiber comes from fruit, vegetables, oats, beans, peas, lentils, and barley. When mixed with liquid, it forms a gel that helps control blood sugar and reduces cholesterol. Insoluble fiber is found in fruits, grains, and vegetables. It adds bulk and acts like a brush to clean out the colon. It helps food pass through the digestive tract more quickly and prevents constipation. A diet rich in fiber can reduce the risk of heart disease, type-2 diabetes, and several forms of cancer. Improvements are also found in cholesterol, blood pressure, and regulation of digestion, all while helping you feel fuller. It is possible to get too much fiber, which can often lead to bloating or more frequent bowel movements. The American Heart Association recommends between 25 and 38 grams of fiber a day in a well-balanced diet. Another method of recommended fiber intake is 10-15 grams per 1000 calories.

HYDRATION

One of the most important responsibilities you have is to supply your body with enough water in order to function. Water is essential in every cellular process in your body. Staying hydrated helps maintain the balance of bodily fluids. The functions of these bodily fluids include digestion, absorption, blood circulation, creation of saliva, transport of nutrients, and maintenance of body temperature. In addition to maintaining the efficiency of bodily functions, drinking enough water can help you feel full and cause you to avoid any second trips for more food. It is recommended to drink at least half a gallon (8 cups) of water a day and additional water depending on physical activity, health condition, and climate. It's beneficial to consume sufficient amounts of water before, during, and after exercise for optimal performance. Common signs that you may need to drink more water include dryness of mouth, headaches, muscle cramping, fatigue, dark-yellow urine, or dizziness. When feeling lazy, tired, or just having an "off-day", sometimes a few cups of water is all you need.

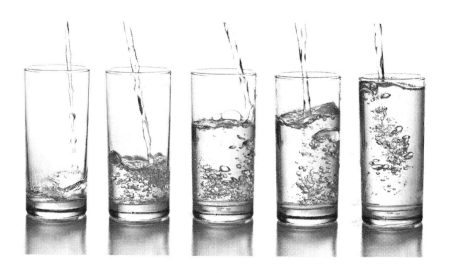

"Life is not about finding yourself. Life is about creating yourself"
~ **Lolly Daskal**

HOW TO READ A NUTRITION FACTS LABEL

You can learn about the contents of a food or drink by looking at the nutrition facts label. The label describes the details of the item including the breakdown of macronutrients and micronutrients.

Nutrition Facts

Serving Size 1/4 Cup (113g)
Servings Per Container 8

Amount Per Serving

Calories 100	Calories from Fat 20

	% Daily Value*
Total Fat 2g	**3%**
Saturated Fat 1.5g	**7%**
Trans Fat 0g	
Cholesterol 10mg	**3%**
Sodium 460mg	**19%**
Total Carbohydrate 4g	**1%**
Dietary Fiber 0g	**0%**
Sugars 4g	
Protein 16g	

Vitamin A 0%	•	Vitamin C 0%
Calcium 8%	•	Iron 0%

* Percent Daily Values are based on a 2,000 calorie diet.

Reading a nutritional label can be easy to understand if you know what information you're interested in. In terms of tracking macros, you're mainly interested in the amount of **total fat**, **total carbohydrates,** and **protein** in each serving. These three macronutrients are the breakdown of **calories**. The nutrients and calories you see on the label are the amounts for the **'serving size'** stated at the top. The amount shown in the parenthesis is a more accurate way of measuring the same serving size. For example, you can measure the serving size on this nutrition label by either '1/4 cup' or '113 grams'.

The **'servings per container'** tell you how many servings there are in the entire product. In this case, there are 8 servings in the container. Towards the bottom of the label you'll find the daily percentage of vitamins and minerals in one serving size. Other information such as the amount of fiber and sodium can also be helpful.

If you are keeping track of fat, protein, and carbs then you are also tracking calories at the same time. Here's how many calories are in one gram of each macronutrient:

- 1g of Fat — **9** calories
- 1g of Carbs— **4** calories
- 1g of Protein — **4** calories

By knowing the amount of grams in each macronutrient you can calculate the total calories. You can do this by multiplying the number of grams in each macronutrient by the number of calories per gram of that macronutrient. Then add the calories from the three macronutrients for the total amount of calories. Using this nutrition label for example:

- Fat: 2g x 9= **18** calories
- Carbs: 4g x 4= **16** calories
- Protein:16g x 4= **64** calories

16 + 64 + 18 = **98** calories

As you see, the 98 calories calculated is a close estimate of the 100 calories shown on the label. Due to rounded numbers, converting grams to calories may not always be exact.

Nutrition Facts

Serving Size 1/4 Cup (113g)
Servings Per Container 8

Amount Per Serving

Calories 100 | Calories from Fat 20

	% Daily Value*
Total Fat 2g	3%
Saturated Fat 1.5g	7%
Trans Fat 0g	
Cholesterol 10mg	3%
Sodium 460mg	19%
Total Carbohydrate 4g	1%
Dietary Fiber 0g	0%
Sugars 4g	
Protein 16g	

Vitamin A 0%	•	Vitamin C 0%
Calcium 8%	•	Iron 0%

* Percent Daily Values are based on a 2,000 calorie diet.

"If you aim at nothing, you will hit it every time" ~ **Zig Ziglar**

TRACKING FOOD

Tracking the food you eat has now become insanely simple and easy to do. With apps such as 'MyFitnessPal', you're able to search and keep track of any food you come across. All you have to do is type the name of the food, set the amount, and you're done. It's even easier to find the exact food or drink by using the barcode scanner. Once you choose the food, you can set the serving size along with how many servings you had. This can all be done in the same amount of time it takes to send a brief text. Tracking your food can be even quicker by saving entire meals in the app so the next time you eat the same thing, it'll be part of your daily food diary within a second.

One might question how to track foods without a nutrition label or any food you haven't prepared yourself. The best way to do so is by estimating the amount of the individual ingredients. For example, a turkey sandwich prepared by someone else can be tracked as two slices of bread, turkey, cheese, mayo, and lettuce. Even though the goal of tracking macros is to be accurate as possible, in most cases it doesn't always have to be perfect. As long as you're within a reasonable range of your macronutrient goals for the day, you will still be making great progress towards reaching your goal. Preparing your own food increases the accuracy of the macros you track since you know exactly how much of the ingredients are in the food you consume.

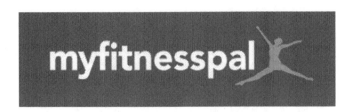

There are many calorie-tracking apps and websites that make the process of losing or gaining weight simple. 'MyFitnessPal' is one of the most popular free apps available due to its wide database of foods and ease of use. By taking advantage of these services, it allows you to make wise food choices that support the progress of your goal. To better understand what you're tracking in 'MyFitnessPal' pay attention to the 'total fat', 'total carbohydrates', and 'protein'. The 'total' column tells you how much of each macronutrient you've had for the day. Knowing how much of each macronutrient you have remaining can help you choose foods that will help you hit your daily goals.

	Total	Goal	Left
Protein	160	194	34g >
Carbohydrates	139	170	31g >
Fiber	17	38	21g >
Sugar	60	73	13g >
Fat	40	54	14g >
Saturated Fat	12	22	10g >
Polyunsaturated Fat	4	N/A	~4g >

Nutrition — Calories — Nutrients — Macros — Day View — Today

"Don't count the days, make the days count" ~ **Muhammad Ali**

FOOD PROFILE

CARBOHYDRATES					
Food	Amount/Size	Calorie	Carb	Fat	Protein
Banana	Medium	105	27	0	1
Blueberries	1 cup	85	21	0.5	1
White Bread	1 slice	70	12	1	4
Wheat Bread	1 slice	70	12	1	4
Broccoli	1 cup	30	6	0	2
Oatmeal	½ cup (dry)	150	27	3	5
Orange Juice	8 fl. oz.	110	26	0	2
Pasta	1 cup (cooked)	220	43	1	8
Potato (White)	Medium	150	33	0	3
Potato (Sweet)	Medium	180	42	0	3
Rice (Brown)	1 cup (cooked)	216	45	2	5
Rice (White)	1 cup (cooked)	206	45	1	4
Yogurt (light)	6 oz.	80	16	0	5
PROTEIN					
Food	Amount/Size	Calorie	Carb	Fat	Protein
Chicken Breast	3 oz. (cooked)	110	0	1	21
Egg	1 large	78	1	5	6
Egg White	1 large	17	0	0	3.5
Milk (Whole)	1 cup	150	12	8	8
Milk (2%)	1 cup	130	12	5	8
Tilapia	3 oz. (cooked)	110	0	2	21
Tuna	1 can (4 oz.)	100	0	1	22
Whey Protein	1 scoop	120	3	1	24
FATS					
Food	Amount/Size	Calorie	Carb	Fat	Protein
Almonds	¼ cup	163	6	14	6
Avocado	1 cup (sliced)	234	12	24	3
Butter	1 tbsp.	70	0	7	0
Cashews	¼ cup	157	9	12	5
Cream Cheese	1 oz.	100	1	10	1
Olive Oil	1 tbsp.	120	0	14	0
Peanut Butter	2 tbsp.	190	7	16	7

SUPPLEMENTS

Most people looking to burn fat or gain muscle immediately turn to supplements as if it is needed to achieve great results. Though supplements can be beneficial, they are only meant to help "supply" your diet and are not needed to reach your goal. Most of the popular supplements can be acquired from food but it can be convenient to have certain ones available. With that said, here are some recommended supplements to aid the pursuit of your fitness goal.

WHEY PROTEIN

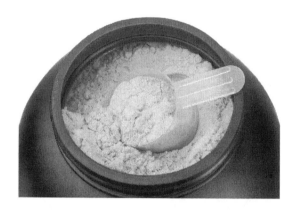

Whey protein is a liquid byproduct of cheese production that is sold as a dietary supplement in the form of powder. It is recognized as a "complete protein" that is fast and easy to digest. A popular measure of protein absorption used is the biological value (BV), in which whey protein has the highest possible value of 100 [2]. With the benefit of quick digestion, consuming whey protein post workout can be *optimal* for muscle growth. Another advantage of whey protein is that it is convenient when food isn't readily available. You can easily mix the powder into a smoothie, oatmeal, or any other recipe. Most people find it challenging to fulfill their daily protein requirement through only food, so consuming whey protein can help you stay consistent with your diet.

CREATINE

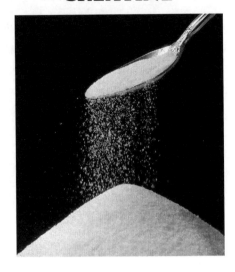

Creatine enhances the body's capacity to perform high intensity work and supports a greater appearance of muscles. Creatine is basically a fuel source for ATP, which is an energy system used for short bursts of power. This strengthens the contraction of muscle fibers and helps an individual achieve more reps. Creatine is found in meat, fish and also in the human body. With many blends of creatine on the market, it is recommended to use the most basic form of the molecule, which is micronized creatine monohydrate. Micronized is essentially creatine monohydrate, but with much smaller molecules making it easier to absorb. The recommended dosage of creatine monohydrate requires 5 grams daily. Any excess amounts will more than likely be excreted without being used since your body is limited to how much it can absorb. This natural molecule has a property that causes water retention in your muscles which produces a more full-muscled appearance. Creatine is also one of the most studied supplements, both in a sports setting and its interactions with various medical conditions. Creatine can be seen as a natural boost to your training performance and an added benefit to the appearance of your muscles.

MULTIVITAMIN

The human body requires a wide variety of vitamins and minerals in order to complete its daily tasks. When living an active lifestyle, your body needs more nutrients than normal to support its activity level. Neglecting these micronutrients can cause your body to work less efficiently, especially when working out. Therefore, it is important to provide your body with the necessary amount of vitamins and minerals for optimal results. Though it is possible to get all of your micronutrients through food only, it can be a challenge to do so each day. Supplementing a multivitamin with your diet will act as a source of insurance in case you don't get enough vitamins and minerals from the food you already consume.

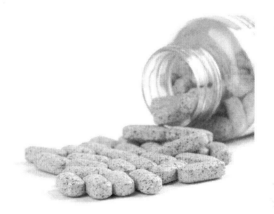

FISH OIL

Fish oil contains essential fatty acids (EFAs) which have been shown to offer endless benefits such as improvements in brain function, cardiovascular and joint health. The two widely researched Omega-3 fatty acids include EPA and DHA which are termed "essential" since we need them for proper function but our bodies cannot produce them. Therefore, we must obtain them through food or supplements. Omega-3 fatty acids work by lowering the body's production of triglycerides. High levels of triglycerides can lead to coronary artery disease, heart disease, and stroke. Studies have shown that benefits of fish oil include a boost in your immune system, anti-inflammatory treatment, improvements in vision, memory, and bone health along with many other advantages. With countless beneficial claims, it serves as smart investment to consume fish oil for overall health.

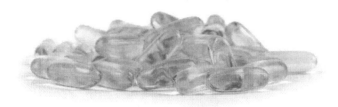

PRE-WORKOUT

Pre-workouts are the least necessary of the recommended supplements. Common ingredients found in a pre-workout supplement include beta-alanine, caffeine, creatine, B vitamins and other performance-based substances. The benefits of a pre-workout vary from increased endurance, more energy, better focus, and greater blood flow to muscles. Consuming a pre-workout can serve as an advantage on the days you feel sluggish and in need of a boost to help get you through your workout. Most pre-workout supplements are consumed before training and usually take about 15-30 minutes to kick in. A common substitute for a pre-workout supplement is caffeine, which has shown to increase training performance on its own.

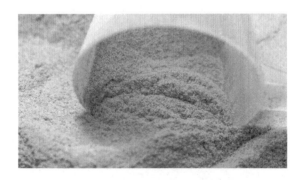

NUTRITION PRIORITY PYRAMID

The purpose of this pyramid is to help clear up any confusion on what aspects of nutrition to consider in terms of achieving your fitness goal. The pyramid starts at the bottom with the most important priority and goes up each stage of lesser importance. It is directed towards the recomposition of your body in terms of building muscle and/or burning fat. With many people training towards their goal, most do not have an idea of the nutritional priorities that will allow them to progress the most. There are individuals who worry about the details of their goal before considering the main points of nutrition that will produce the results they're looking for. One might ask, "Should I drink 2% milk or whole milk?" without knowing the factors that need to be considered in order to accurately answer that question. Information such as the person's fitness goal, macronutrient requirements, and other deciding factors need to be acknowledged before providing a legitimate answer. When in doubt about your nutritional priorities, turn to this pyramid for better assurance. Credit for the idea of this pyramid goes to Eric Helms, a coach at '3DMuscleJourney'.

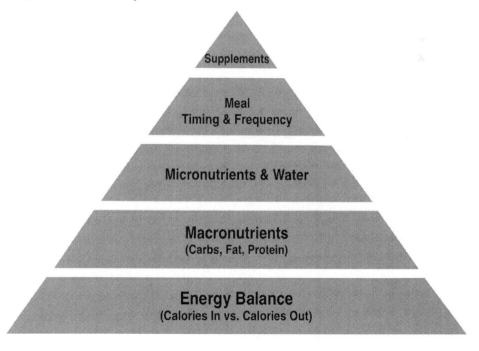

1. ENERGY BALANCE

The most important aspect of recomposing your physique is the balance of the calories you consume (food/drinks) and the calories your body uses (physical activity). These two factors ultimately decide what will happen to your bodyweight over time. You can gain, lose, or maintain your weight depending on how you balance your calories. If the amount of calories coming into your body is equal to the amount of calories coming out, then you will remain the same weight. If the amount of calories coming in is more than the amount coming out, you will gain weight. Lastly, if the amount of calories coming in is less than the amount coming out then this will result in you losing weight.

In order to have the right energy balance (caloric balance) you need to know the amount of calories you need to achieve your specific goal. To determine the amount, it is common to start by calculating the amount of calories your body will need just to maintain its weight. Factors that will determine this caloric amount include age, height, weight, sex, and level of physical activity. The amount that is generated from these factors is a good estimate of how many calories your body requires to stay at its current weight (the actual amount of calories you require is determined by how your body metabolizes the food you consume). Once you know the amount of calories it takes to maintain your weight, you will either lower the amount of calories to support weight loss or increase the calories for weight gain. The amount by which your calories are adjusted will determine how fast or slow your weight will change. The rate at which your weight changes may affect how much muscle mass you maintain while in a caloric deficit and how much fat you gain when in a caloric surplus.

If you don't know how many calories you are feeding your body, it is hard to control your energy balance. You don't want to be disappointed from the lack of results because you didn't have your energy balance in check. So knowing whether you are in a caloric deficit, surplus, or maintenance is the most important priority when trying to change the composition of your body.

2. MACRONUTRIENTS

Once your energy balance is in check, it is now important to know where these calories are coming from. Calories are made up of three macronutrients, which include fats, protein, and carbs. It is beneficial to know how much of these macronutrients we consume in our diet. For example, one's diet may consist of 40% protein, 40% carbs, and 20% fat. The amount of macronutrients can also be evaluated in terms of grams instead of percentages. Different proportions will have an impact on how the body changes and feels. Even if you consume the same amount of calories, adjusting the proportion of macronutrients can cause your body to change its composition. It is likely to increase protein while decreasing carbs for fat loss, and to consume a moderate amount of protein while increasing carbs for weight gain. Different ratios of fats, protein, and carbs will be *optimal* for specific goals, so it can be beneficial to have an experienced coach who can create a personalized plan for you. More on information on the importance of macronutrients and how they affect your body is in the 'Why Track Macros' section.

3. MICRONUTRIENTS AND WATER

Although the amount of macronutrients you consume has a major impact on the composition of your body, micronutrients are just as important. Progress towards your fitness goal can be affected if vitamins and minerals are neglected. Micronutrients help maintain a healthy-functioning body and support the metabolism of fats, protein, and carbs. High amounts of vitamins and minerals can be found in fruits and vegetables. General recommendations include at least a serving of fruits and vegetables per 1000 calories. So if an individual consumes 2000 calories per day, then they should consume at least 2 servings of fruits and 2 servings of vegetables. Consuming a wide variety of whole foods will help ensure that you are getting enough vitamins and minerals. More on the importance of vitamins and minerals are discussed in the 'Vitamins and Minerals' section.

Water consumption is extremely important in reaching any fitness goal. Water is involved in every bodily function, so insufficient hydration can affect the way your body feels and operates. Frequent clear urinations throughout the day are good indicators to whether you are drinking enough water. Most people usually don't have an issue with drinking more water while achieving their fitness goal, so this isn't a priority that has to be monitored as closely as the previous two stages. The 'Hydration' section includes more information on the importance of drinking water.

4. MEAL TIMING AND FREQUENCY

Meal timing and frequency does not make a huge difference in terms of fat loss or muscle gain but it can beneficial if implemented properly. Your balance of calories and macronutrients will ultimately determine any changes in your body composition. The benefits of meal timing are directed more toward how you feel throughout the day and your energy while training. It makes sense to consume carbs 1-2 hours before your workout so you have enough energy to train even though some people do well without eating anything beforehand.

Consuming meals at specific times is more of a preference than something you have to do in order to burn fat or build muscle. Having 3-5 meals a day is recommended but as long as the required calories are met at the end of the day, the outcome of fat loss and muscle growth will relatively be the same. In order to maximize the theoretical benefits of building muscle, it is best to spread your total amount of protein throughout the day. Several studies have shown that consuming protein and carbs post workout is beneficial for *optimal* muscle recovery. As you plan the timing of your meals, it is helpful to consider the regulation of glucose and levels of hunger. The main points of the day to consume carbs are in the morning, pre and post workout. A simple rule of thumb when it comes to meal frequency is to "eat when you're hungry". More details on meal timing and frequency are explained in the '6 Meals A Day' section of 'Common Misconceptions'.

5. SUPPLEMENTS

This is the least important stage of the priority pyramid. Supplements are beneficial for whatever you can't already get from actual food. The word itself explains that is it supplementary, meaning it is intended to supply your diet. For example, an individual may have a hard time getting all their protein from only food, which would make sense to supplement with whey protein in order to help fulfill their protein requirement. You shouldn't rely on supplements over food as the foundation of your nutrition. This is where most people go wrong because they feel that there is something special in supplement jars that will allow them to bypass good nutrition to attain their desired results. Yet these individuals may achieve little to no progress because they neglected the more important aspects of their nutrition. When choosing a supplement, you should always do your own research on the product and check reviews to help you decide whether it will have a significant impact on the results you're looking for. Some supplements are unnecessary while pursuing specific goals so pay attention to the quality and how effective the product would be for you. The *'Supplements'* section explains which supplements are most beneficial for achieving certain results.

6. LIFESTYLE & BEHAVIOR

This topic is not displayed as a stage in the pyramid but rather revolves around it and should be considered at all levels. While prioritizing your nutrition and training, keep in mind that the reality of pursuing your goal should be sustainable and not life controlling. There are some people who quit too soon because they don't enjoy their diets and feel too restricted. Then there are others who are over-achievers and try to be perfect with every aspect of achieving their goal. With many individuals pursuing their goals, remember that being happy, positive and enjoying life is part of being fit. With a wide variety of food in the world, everyone should be allowed to enjoy what they like to eat no matter what their goal is. Being able to enjoy the foods you love allows you to be more flexible and dedicated to your diet. Limiting yourself while missing out on the foods you really like isn't sustainable over a lifetime. Every individual should be able to eat out within reason and thanks to the calorie-awareness apps such as 'MyFitnessPal' you can easily search the amount of nutrients in almost any food there is.

You don't have to stress yourself out about the thought of hitting your calories or macros every single day in order to see great results. Understanding the relationship between what you consume and your body's daily allowance, serves you more control, flexibility, and confidence when enjoying the food and drinks you love. It is likely that you will confront temptations or certain situations that can steer you away from your diet, but these occasional mishaps will not dictate your results as long as consistency is kept towards your goal. Though it is important to resist temptations and be consistent as possible, trying to do so shouldn't take over your life. While pursuing any fitness goal, focus on keeping an overall balance that will allow you to maintain a healthy lifestyle.

II. OPTIMAL TRAINING

"Opportunities are sometimes disguised as hard work,
so most people don't recognize them"
~ Ann Landers

MUSCLE GROUPS

The body is categorized into several muscle groups, which include the **chest, back, shoulders, legs, biceps, triceps,** and **abdominals.** The legs are generally made up of the quadriceps, hamstrings, and calves, while also including the glutes in most of its exercises. The shoulders are made up of the upper traps and deltoids (delts). The deltoid has three main muscles that include the front, lateral, and rear delt. The biceps are made up of two main heads, hence the term "bi", while the triceps contain three heads. The back generally consists of the lats, an upper, middle, and lower back. Some muscle groups work together during certain exercises. For example, the flat bench press primarily focuses on the chest while the triceps and shoulders help to complete the movement. Understanding which muscles are stimulated during specific exercises can allow you to set up an efficient workout that will target your goal.

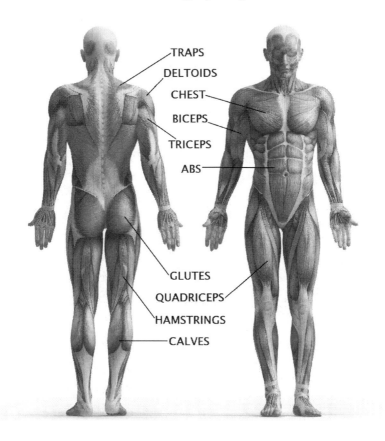

TRAPS
DELTOIDS
CHEST
BICEPS
TRICEPS
ABS
GLUTES
QUADRICEPS
HAMSTRINGS
CALVES

HOW DO MUSCLES GROW?

Lifting weights damages your muscles. Though that may sound strange, pumping iron at the gym actually depletes muscle-building nutrients in your body and creates microscopic tears in your muscle fibers. It is only until after your workout that your body begins to repair the damage you inflicted on it and you experience the muscle growth you desire [3]. An effective workout results in minimal bleeding and tearing of your muscle fibers, which often leads to soreness. This damage is an essential part of building muscle and indicates that your muscles are repairing and becoming stronger. Muscle repair usually takes at least two days, making 48 hours of rest essential for *optimal* growth.

The principle behind muscle growth is known as progressive overload. It states that you must impose a demand on your muscles greater than what they're accustomed to. Your muscles compensate for this strain on a cellular level by adding protein to grow thicker and stronger. Once your muscle adapts to the load by becoming stronger, a progressive overload such as more weight or reps must be added for more growth. Overall, muscle damage takes place during the workout, and repair and growth happens when you are at rest.

"If there is no struggle, there is no progress" ~ Frederick Douglass

CHOOSING AN EXERCISE

By sticking to basic exercises, you can build a solid foundation of muscle. Compound movements such as the squat, bench press, and deadlift are great because they stimulate multiple muscle groups while burning relatively more calories. Isolation exercises such as the bicep curl or leg extension focuses on one specific muscle group. Both compound and isolation exercises are good to incorporate in your workout. A variety of exercises should be used in order to engage all areas of the muscle group. By using effective exercises to target different angles on the muscle, you will develop a more detailed and defined physique.

WEIGHT TRAINING EXERCISES

Chest (Compound chest exercises also target the triceps and shoulders secondarily)	• Flat Barbell or Dumbbell Bench Press* • Incline Barbell or Dumbbell Bench Press* • Decline Barbell or Dumbbell Bench Press • Flat Chest Press Machine • Incline Chest Press Machine* • Decline Chest Press Machine • Dips • Push-Ups* • Flat/Incline/Decline Dumbbell Fly • Pec Deck Machine* • Cable Crossovers/Cable Fly* • Dumbbell Pullover
Back (Compound back exercises also target the biceps secondarily)	• Pull-Ups* • Chin-Ups • Lat Pull-Down* • Bent Over Barbell Row* • Dumbbell Row* • T-Bar Row • Seated Cable Row • Chest Supported Machine Row*
Shoulders (Compound shoulder exercises also target the triceps secondarily)	• Overhead Barbell or Dumbbell Press • Overhead Machine Press • Arnold Press • Dumbbell or Barbell Upright Rows* • Dumbbell or Cable Lateral Raises* • Dumbbell or Cable Front Raises* • Dumbbell or Cable Rear Delt Rows* • Machine Rear Delt Fly • Dumbbell, Barbell or Machine Shrugs
Quadriceps (Compound quad exercises also target a significant portion of the lower body/posterior chain)	• Squats* • Front Squats • Barbell or Dumbbell Lunges • Barbell or Dumbbell Step-Ups • Leg Press* • Machine Squat or Hack Squat • Leg Extensions*

43

Hamstrings (Compound hamstring exercises also target a significant portion of the lower body/posterior chain)	• Romanian Deadlifts* • Dumbbell Straight Leg Deadlifts* • Dumbbell Sumo Deadlifts • Squats • Glute-Ham Raises • Hyperextensions • Cable Pull-Through • Good-Mornings • Leg Curls*
Biceps	• Barbell Curls* • Dumbbell Curls* • Barbell or Dumbbell Preacher Curls • Seated Dumbbell Curls • Hammer Curls* • Concentration Curls • Cable Curls* • Biceps Curl Machine
Triceps	• Dips • Flat Close Grip Bench Press • Decline Close Grip Bench Press • Close Grip Push-Ups • Skull Crushers* • Overhead Dumbbell Triceps Extensions* • Cable Press-Downs* • Bench Dips*
Abs	• Decline Bench Sit-ups* • Oblique V-Ups* • Bench Knee Tucks* • Ab Wheel Rollout* • Crunches • Leg Raises • Russian Twist • Plank • Hanging Knee Raises*
Calves	• Seated Dumbbell Calve Raises* • Standing Dumbbell Calves Raises* • Leg Press Calf Raises

*Frequently used by the author   [4]

HOW TO WARM-UP

A full warm-up consists of three stages. The first stage involves raising your body temperature to prepare for the intensity of physical activity. Doing 5-10 minutes of cardio exercise such as jogging, biking, jumping jacks, or an elliptical machine should be sufficient to get the job done. Second, is to stretch and work on the mobility of your muscles and joints. Another 5-10 minutes of various stretching exercises will prepare your muscles to handle resistance and help prevent injury. A full body stretch isn't always necessary but can be helpful. Mobility is the ability to move freely and easily. Mobility exercises are beneficial for preventing injury and allows for full range of motion during training. Lastly, you should prepare the muscle for weight training by starting your workout with fairly light weight. Gradually increasing the weight at the start of an exercise prepares the muscle to handle heavier loads while allowing you to grasp a better feel for the movement. Neglecting a proper warm-up can limit your performance, increase the risk of injury, and result in being excessively tight or sore post-workout.

HOW MUCH WEIGHT?

The weight you choose for an exercise should suit the amount of reps you plan to do without sacrificing good form. Most people pick a weight that is too heavy and end up using bad form, which can produce inefficient results and often lead to injury. Some individuals use a weight that is too light, which can make it difficult to stimulate growth in the muscle. Overall, choose a desired rep range, and then pick a weight that will challenge you for the set amount of reps. When trying a new exercise, you should use a relatively light weight until you understand how to perform the movement correctly. Once you feel comfortable with the form, then increase the weight until it is challenging to complete the required amount of reps. As you get stronger and able to perform more reps at this weight, you will eventually need to increase the load. Using the heaviest weight for an exercise isn't always the best option. Even though you may be able to do 1-2 reps for an exercise, using a lighter weight that will allow you to complete more reps can produce more muscle development.

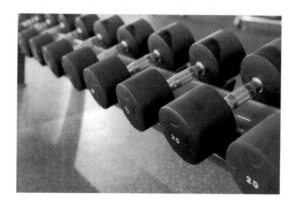

HOW MANY REPS AND SETS?

A repetition is a single execution of any exercise. If you do a set of 10 bicep curls consecutively, then that's 10 repetitions. The amount of reps you choose typically determines your training style. You can train for muscular endurance, strength, or a combination of both. The high rep range (12-20) supports muscular endurance training while the lower rep range (3-8) is focused more on strength. To train your muscles for both strength and endurance, the two rep ranges are compromised at an ideal range of 8-12 reps. You may often have to adjust the weight to fit your desired rep range. For example, if you're training for strength and endurance and can't complete eight reps, then the weight may be too heavy. If you can do more than 12 reps, then the weight is too light. With trial and error, you'll eventually find a weight that challenges you within that rep range.

Training till 'failure' is when you cannot complete another rep with good form. In other words, this is the point during an exercise where you have to sacrifice good form in order to perform one more rep. Though you don't have to train to failure in order for muscles to grow, you should come close. A good target for most of your sets is to perform the exercise until you are 1-2 reps away from failure. Training till you reach failure can significantly fatigue your muscles and should only be used towards the end of your sets or workout. Though training to failure should only be used occasionally throughout the workout, you don't have to limit your sets to a specific number of reps. If you've reached your target number of reps during a set and you are able to perform 1-2 more reps with good form, then do so within reason. The last few reps will be the deciding factor to whether or not you stimulate growth in your muscle.

A set is a combination of consistent reps of a single exercise. You generally want to do 1-2 warm up sets with a lighter weight for each exercise before moving on to heavier sets. Although there is no specific amount of sets that an individual should do, the total sets per exercise typically range from 3-5. You want to allow yourself enough sets to effectively stimulate the muscle to grow. It's beneficial to incorporate a moderate amount of sets per exercise to allow time and energy for other exercises in the workout.

REST PERIOD BETWEEN SETS

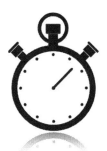

The amount of rest you take in between your sets has a major impact on the quality and intensity of your training. Many people wait too long to start their next set, which can hinder the productivity of their training. Once you finish a set of a particular exercise, you've achieved a blood pump into the muscle. Maintaining this temporary pump is a key advantage to building new muscle. The longer you wait to start the next set is the more likely that this pump will go away. On the other hand, resting too little can quickly fatigue the muscle and affect the overall efficiency of the workout. The idea is to give your muscles enough time to slightly recover while keeping the rest time short enough to challenge its ability to perform. The amount of rest time you should allow yourself depends on whether you want to train for strength, muscle growth, or endurance. Though these training styles are relatively dependent upon one another, you can directly target each one by controlling the rest time in between sets. It is recommended to take 3-5 minutes of rest when training for strength, 1-2 minutes for muscle growth, and 45- 90 seconds for endurance. Compound exercises can be more exhausting and may require more rest since they involve the use of multiple muscle groups. Rest periods can also vary among individuals. It can take 30 seconds for an individual to fully recover from a working set while someone else may need 60 seconds. The key is to find the thin line between taking too much and too little rest for the benefit of achieving *optimal* results.

TRAINING VOLUME

Training volume is a combination of sets, reps, and weight. Each of these factors has a direct effect on the total volume. Whether you like to train heavy or light, it's always possible to achieve the same training volume by varying the sets, weights, or reps. For example, 1 set of 20 reps with a 50lb weight (1 x 20 x 50 =1000) is equal to 1 set of 10 reps with a 100lb weight (1 x 10 x 100 =1000). As shown, you can vary the reps, weight, and sets to fit your style of training while controlling the total volume of your workout. While other factors such as the amount of rest between sets will determine the intensity of a workout, volume serves as a representation of how much work is done.

PROPER FORM

Performing an exercise correctly is one of the most important aspects of building a great physique. By using proper form, it allows you to fully target and develop your muscles while minimizing the risk of injury. Some individuals use momentum and cheat proper form for the sake of training with a heavy weight. It is far more beneficial to use a weight that allows you to perform an exercise properly than to sacrifice form just to use a heavier weight. The key to building muscle is not how heavy you can lift but rather how much damage you can inflict on the muscle in order to stimulate growth. Using proper form also allows a person to develop a greater mind-muscle connection during the exercise. This connection incorporates the thought of contracting the intended muscle in an exercise to better engage it throughout the movement. The better you are able to use the muscle to control the weight is the more development you can achieve. An improvement in the use of proper form is a sign of progress in your training. Therefore, taking the time to learn how to perform an exercise correctly is extremely beneficial towards building muscle and strength.

SIGNS THAT YOU ARE MAKING PROGRESS IN YOUR TRAINING

Being able to lift a heavier weight is often seen as the only sign that your training has improved. Though being able to push more weight is a good sign, it is only a fraction of many observations that can confirm you've made progress in your training. Other signs include the ability to complete more reps, shorter rest time, and an improvement in form. For example, if you were able to squat a certain amount of weight for 8 reps last week and this week you're able to complete 9 reps using the same weight, then that extra rep is an obvious sign of progress. What if we can make progress without changing the amount of weight or reps? By shortening the amount of rest in between sets, you allow yourself less time to recover making it a greater challenge on the muscle to perform. If you are able to complete the same workout while resting for shorter periods, then you've made progress in your training.

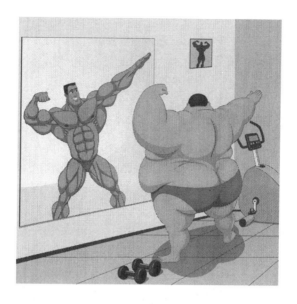

One sign of improvement that is often overlooked is the ability to perform an exercise using proper form. Focusing on maintaining good form as the set gets tough, challenges your muscles just as much as adding weight or doing more reps. Completing the same workout with the use of better form is another sure sign of progress in your training. By following a consistent routine, improvements in your training will become more noticeable. Your body does not want to change its current condition so it will take time to see significant results. It is fine if a week or two goes by without noticing any progress but with patience, consistency, and hard work you will eventually see the results you've been training for. Progress in training can be a result of building muscle, strength, endurance, or becoming mentally tougher. No matter what kind of improvement is made, any one of them will surely bring you closer to achieving your fitness goal.

"To understand the heart and mind of a person, look not at what he has already achieved, but at what he aspires to do" ~ Khalil Gibran

CENTRAL NERVOUS SYSTEM

The central nervous system consists of the brain, spinal cord, and a complex network of neurons. This system is responsible for sending, receiving, and interpreting information throughout all parts of the body. Your CNS controls every thought and movement in the body, making it extremely important to maintain its health. Extensive training without sufficient rest increases the risk of damage to your CNS. Most cells in your CNS cannot be repaired or renewed and can lose some of its abilities. Signs of damage include difficulty with physical activity, recovering, comprehending information, and other symptoms. The CNS is at an increased risk for damage while consuming fewer calories than normal, which emphasizes the need for sufficient nutrients and recovery while dieting. Just like the muscular system, your CNS can be overworked. Yet with proper nutrition and efficient training you can protect and maintain the health of your central nervous system.

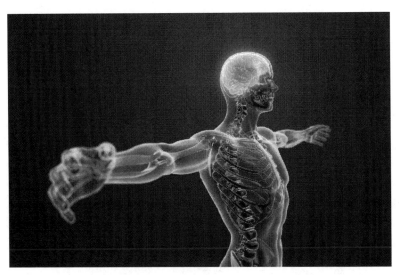

The CNS is made up of the brain and spinal cord

REST DAY

It is important to occasionally incorporate a full day of rest from training in order to allow your body sufficient recovery. As training becomes more frequent, your body is at greater risk for injury due to strain on muscles, tendons, ligaments, bones and joints. Muscle fibers are broken down during weight training, so sufficient time is needed for the body to repair and grow new muscle. It can be smart to train certain muscles on specific days so you can allow other muscles to recover. For example, training upper body on one day and lower body on a separate day, allows one muscle group to recover while training another. Benefits of incorporating a rest day include improvements in training performance, a stronger immune system, and more energy. If desired, you can remain active during a rest day with light exercise such as jogging, yoga, or stretching.

"Patience is also a form of action" ~ **Auguste Rodin**

HOW FREQUENT SHOULD YOU TRAIN?

The frequency of your training should depend on the intensity of your workouts and your physical ability. The intensity of your workout is one of the main factors that determine how much stress you are putting on your body. Training at a low intensity will allow you to exercise more frequently compared to training with high intensity. The individual's physical ability also has an impact on how frequent they should train. For example, an athletic person may be comfortable training at a high intensity 6-7 days a week while someone fairly new to working out should start training at the same level of intensity no more than 3-4 days a week. Your workout schedule should be attainable and aligned with your fitness goal.

An individual's training schedule should also correspond with how their body recovers. Some muscles recover faster or slower than others, so knowing how your body responds to training can help you efficiently plan your workouts. Muscles require a minimum of 48 hours to fully recover from a workout, so you should avoid training the same muscle group everyday to allow *optimal* growth. Proper rest and nutrients are needed before you can train the same muscle group again. A general rule of thumb is 'if you're still sore, you're not ready to train that body part again'. An individual should also be aware of protecting the health of their central nervous system. Even though a person may have the energy to train at a high intensity every day, your CNS can be affected. With several factors to consider in training frequency, you should work out as much as you desire while monitoring your overall health.

10 COMMON TRAINING MISTAKES

1. LIFTING TOO HEAVY

Using more weight doesn't always equal a better workout. Letting go of your ego can allow you to grow more muscle. It's best to engage the muscle as much as possible and by using too much weight it is likely that you would have to use bad form in order to complete the exercise. It is better to use a moderate weight that you can control through the entire movement, then work your way up to a heavier weight that you can properly control.

2. IMPROPER TECHNIQUE

Some people never seek the benefits of their training because they consistently use bad form. An individual can do 20 "bicep curls" and barely work their muscle because of using improper form. By using small techniques such as how to eliminate momentum and using the target muscle to control the weight, your workouts will become more productive. Using the correct form will also reduce your risk of injury.

3. NOT ENOUGH RESEARCH BEFORE COMING TO THE GYM

There are some individuals who come to the gym and watch others work out in hopes of finding an idea of what to do. Starting your workout without a plan can limit your progress and waste valuable time. Your training can become more efficient and flexible by doing research on workouts, proper exercise techniques, and general tips on training. Use the resources that I've posted in the *Resources to Maximize Your Fitness Potential* section for online fitness advice.

4. UNREALISTIC EXPECTATIONS

Expecting to achieve your greatest physique in a few days can be unrealistic. Your body needs time to change. It may take weeks or even months based on your current condition before you can achieve the physique you desire. The main thing is to be patient and focus on progressing one day at a time.

5. RESTING TOO LONG

While everyone needs to rest in between sets, most individuals give themselves too long of a rest period. Some people end up texting or talking, allowing their body too much time to relax. Consistently resting for too long can negatively affect the results of your workout. The key is to limit the time in between sets to challenge your body to become stronger.

6. DOUBTING YOURSELF

Negative thoughts can affect your training performance. By staying positive you allow yourself to have a better workout. Keep in mind that you have no choice but to make progress whenever you try something new. Stay focused and believe that you can accomplish your goals.

7. TRYING TO DO TOO MUCH AT ONCE

Doing cardio, lifting weights, eating healthy, drinking more water, timing your meals and getting more sleep are only some of the many aspects of fitness to improve on. Trying to do everything at once can be challenging for most individuals. It is better to take small steps towards your fitness goal rather than one huge transition that can be difficult to maintain.

8. NOT EATING ENOUGH

Eating healthier is a great start to becoming fit and can cause a diet to be lower in calories. Yet consuming too little calories in addition to training can cause an individual to feel sluggish. Though some people may be cutting back on calories to burn fat, it is important to still fuel your body with enough calories to support energy throughout the day. By properly setting up your macros, you can maximize the amount of calories you are able to consume while achieving your goal.

9. LACK OF VARIETY IN EXERCISES

Incorporating a variety of exercises in your workout is important for developing a well-rounded physique. Understanding which muscles are engaged during specific exercises can allow your workouts to become more efficient. For example, your legs are made up of different muscle groups, so choosing an exercise to target each area is beneficial for overall muscle development.

10. NOT WARMING UP

Before starting a workout and giving it all you've got, it's important to properly prepare your body to efficiently manage the impact of training. Warming up allows the body to gradually adjust to high levels of physical activity, which reduces the risk of injury and improves training performance.

TRAINING MENTALITY

Focus. This is the main difference between training and just working out. "Working out" consists of simply doing exercises without a specific goal in mind. "Training" demands that you exercise with greater principles that not only make you physically stronger, but also mentally tougher as well. Your mentality is the deciding factor that sets you apart from your intentions to train or to just simply work out. An individual who trains pushes through the every set and does not give up just because they feel the burn. The pain of fighting through a set is only temporary, yet will leave you physically and mentally stronger. Your characteristics are a reflection of your mentality, so staying dedicated to your workout can strengthen your self-discipline.

A person who wants to train comes to the gym with a plan so they don't have to worry about what to do once they get there. You should plan the muscle groups, exercises, sets, and rep ranges you want to work on so you have nothing else to do but focus on completing the workout. Even a bad plan is better than having no plan at all. One who comes to train isn't worried about anyone else in the gym. Never feel embarrassed about other people watching as you train. If there is anyone that should feel ashamed, it should be the person watching since they should be training as well. Your focus should be on performing each exercise in the workout to the best of your ability.

Focus on doing better than your last workout. The outcome of whether you're able to successfully increase the weight or reps in your workout depends on your state of mind. The body follows what the mind thinks, so mentally push through your workouts for the result of a greater physique. Instead of hoping your muscles grow, force it to grow by pushing past your limits. Think of each workout as making you 1% stronger and through consistent training your fitness goal is guaranteed. Your training mentality carries over into other aspects of your life so strengthening your mindset during training will help improve other weak points. Most people only see the physical benefits of training but in order to produce significant changes in your physique, it starts with your mentality.

III. OPTIMAL FITNESS THEORY

"Life isn't about waiting for the storm to pass, it's about learning how to dance in the f**king rain" ~ Greg Plitt

COMMON FITNESS MISCONCEPTIONS

The world of fitness is filled with convincing theories that claim to help you reach your goals. Some are beneficial while others can take you down a road of unnecessary effort and misleading results. This section tackles the most popular misconceptions when using nutrition and training to achieve your desired physique.

MISCONCEPTION #1: CARDIO TO LOSE WEIGHT

You often see people running tons of miles on the treadmill in hopes of losing weight. Although cardio improves general health, it is not necessary in order to burn fat. Cardio exercises such as running, biking, and the elliptical machine are all tools to help aide weight loss, but the deciding factor to whether your weight changes is your body's balance of calories. Cardio can be a waste of time if your diet isn't in check. For example, an individual can run 10 miles that burns 1,000 calories, then eat 1,500 calories and result in gaining weight. Weight loss is best executed by controlling your diet. A banana is generally 100 calories, and it takes approximately 100 calories to run 1 mile. So would it be easier to run a mile or simply not eat a banana? Unless you're a monkey and fantasize over bananas, it would most likely be easier to avoid running a mile. This is a prime example of being smarter about reaching your goal, instead of unnecessarily overworking yourself.

Once your diet is in check, you can then consider cardio to burn more calories. While cardio supports weight loss, doing too much may often present a flat appearance in your muscles. Weight training on the other hand develops your muscles, which adds more detail to your physique. Use your calories for the exercises that will develop the kind of results you want. Although you can acquire a great physique without the use of cardio, it is beneficial under certain conditions. It can be a challenge to provide your body with enough nutrients while following a low-calorie diet. Therefore, cardio is useful for burning additional calories, which can allow you to avoid lowering the amount of calories you consume while trying to lose fat.

MISCONCEPTION #2: TONING

In order to acquire a "toned" look that most people desire, an individual must either lower their body fat or build more muscle. By doing both, you can define your physique even quicker. You can only make your muscles bigger or smaller, and you can only gain or lose fat. Fat cannot turn into muscle, nor can muscle turn into fat. Decreasing your body fat percentage requires you to burn more calories than you consume. In order to build muscle you must challenge your muscles enough to grow through the use of exercise. Some people often desire to stay the same weight while achieving a toned physique. Since a pound of muscle is denser than a pound of fat, it is possible to acquire a more defined physique while weighing the same. Muscles take a lot longer to grow than it takes to lose fat. Therefore, your weight will most likely decrease due to the loss of fat when achieving these results in a short period of time.

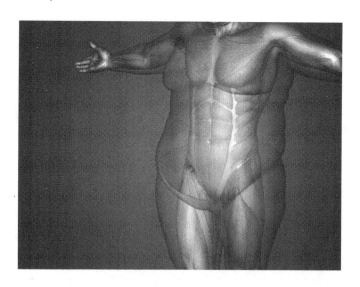

"The only place success comes before work is in the dictionary"
~ Vince Lombardi

MISCONCEPTION #3: TARGETING FAT LOSS

Some individuals desire to lose fat only in their stomach, legs, or some other part of their body. Targeting the reduction of fat in a specific area on your body is not possible. The areas in which you lose and gain fat are already predetermined by your genetics. Some areas of fat on your body will take longer to go away than others. For example, an individual can lose most of the fat on their arms while holding a lot of fat around their stomach. The lower stomach is commonly one of the more difficult areas to lose fat. In order to burn fat in that stubborn area you will just have to continue dieting. Eventually the body will decide to burn fat in the stubborn areas once it reaches a lower percentage of body fat. There is no workout or substance that will allow you to burn fat in one specific area of your body.

MISCONCEPTION #4: AB-TRAINING

Some people believe that in order to have amazing abs, you have to train them hard every day. The abdominal muscles need time to recover just like other muscles on your body, so training them everyday isn't necessary. Abs best respond to high reps and short rest periods in between sets. Implementing additional weight in your ab training will help to develop more mass. Ensure that you choose exercises that will target each section of the abdominals including the upper, lower, and oblique areas. It is important to remember that your body fat percentage must be low enough to see your abs. You can train your abs enough to grow, but if you have a thick layer of fat over the muscle, then they will not be visible.

MISCONCEPTION #5: EATING JUNK FOOD

Eating junk food doesn't have to get in the way of achieving your fitness goal. The more you know about how your body handles food, is the less guilt you will feel about what you consume. Anything you eat or drink will be broken down into a carbohydrate, fat, or protein. So even if you eat a cheeseburger, but you are still within your macronutrient goals for the day, then you will not interrupt the progress of losing fat or building muscle.

With the IIFYM (If It Fits Your Macros) method of losing weight, people often get confused into thinking you should eat as much junk food you want as long as it fits into your macronutrient goals. Even though doing so can allow you to achieve your desired physique, your internal health will be at risk. Before committing yourself to a cheeseburger or milkshake, be sure that you are getting most of your nutrients from whole foods each day.

MISCONCEPTION #6: ALCOHOL

Most people are afraid to drink alcoholic beverages in fear that it will ruin the progress towards their fitness goal. It is fine to have some alcohol as long as it is in moderation. Alcohol has calories (7 calories per gram), so knowing the amount in the drink and how many calories you are allowed will help you stay on pace for achieving your fitness goal. You can substitute the calories from drinking for a portion of fat or carbs on that day, yet be sure you're getting enough healthy nutrients from food since alcohol will not provide any. Implementing cardio or extra physical activity in your schedule can help burn additional calories to allow room for a drink or two. It is helpful to consume lots of water beforehand to prevent dehydration and excess drinking. Having an occasional wine or beer will not ruin your progress as long as you are able to fit it into a healthy diet.

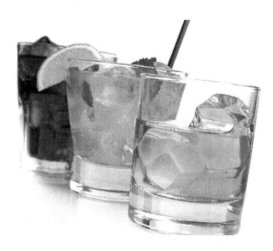

MISCONCEPTION #7: TOO MUCH SUGAR

It is true that consuming too much sugar can lead to long-term health risks such as diabetes, organ failure, and several diseases. Yet in terms of fat loss, eating large amounts of sugar will not prevent you from losing weight as long as the required calories to burn fat are met over time. All carbohydrates are eventually broken down to sugar once digested in your body. Some food sources such as complex carbs take longer to break down while others are already in a simple form such as pure sugar. Since your body uses carbs as a primary source of fuel during physical activity, the more active you are is the more carbs you are allowed. Individuals who burn lots of calories can get away with consuming more sugar since it is being utilized instead of accumulating in the body.

Sugar has a bad rap because it is easy to overeat. Just as everything else, having too much of anything can be bad for you. Consuming whole foods, which are more nutritious and filling will help to regulate the overall consumption of sugar. In terms of losing fat, substituting sweet foods such as raw honey or agave nectar for pure sugar is insignificant since they still contain simple carbs which break down to sugar in your body. Sweeteners such as 'Equal', 'Splenda', or stevia will however make a difference since they contain zero calories. Understanding how many carbs you are allowed will help you to know how much sugar you are able to consume while pursuing your fitness goal.

MISCONCEPTION #8: TOO MUCH SODIUM

Prioritizing your salt intake has an insignificant role in burning fat or building muscle. This is more of a precaution to your general health rather a necessity to building a great physique. Regulating levels of sodium can help lower blood pressure, while decreasing the risks of heart disease and stroke. When sodium is in the body it binds to water and maintains the balance of fluids. It also works together with potassium to help maintain electrical processes across cell membranes, which is critical for nerve transmission, muscular contraction, and other various functions. The body cannot function without sodium, so limiting your intake without any regard to how much you actually need, can be a potential risk.

An increase in sodium causes the body to hold more water, which is a reason why your bodyweight fluctuates throughout the day. Reducing sodium intake helps to lower body weight but is mainly due to the temporary loss of water. It is important to keep in mind that in most cases the goal is not to lose water but to burn fat. There are important times to monitor sodium intake such as when preparing for a bodybuilding competition or photo shoot. Bodybuilders or models may manipulate their salt intake to give their physique a dry, skin-tight appeal when they are already lean enough to see the detail of their muscles.

MISCONCEPTION #9: METABOLISM

People often use their metabolism as an excuse for why they haven't achieved their fitness goal. Others claim that eating certain foods will boost their metabolism and cause them to lose weight. As the term metabolism finds its way into misleading theories each day, it is a "gray" area for most people and can use some clarification. Metabolism is simply how much food your body can process in a day. It is the process by which your body converts what you eat and drink into energy that your body can use. The speed of your metabolism or basal metabolic rate (BMR) determines how many calories your body will require in order to function. Several factors that influence your BMR include your body size, sex, and age.

For the most part, your body's energy requirement to process food stays relatively steady and isn't easily changed[5]. Therefore it is insignificant to rely on certain foods to boost your metabolism in order to lose weight. Your body is designed for you to fulfill the amount of calories needed to support your metabolism by telling you that you're hungry when you need more calories, and to stop eating when you have enough calories. Having a "slow" metabolism simply means your body requires less calories than the average person with your body specifications, while having a "fast" metabolism allows you to consume more. If you feel that you have a slow metabolism and you want to eat more food without gaining weight, then you can increase your body's caloric requirement for the day by burning more calories through physical activity. Whether you have a slow or fast metabolism, it is important to figure out how many calories your body needs to support your weight and plan your fitness goal around that amount.

MISCONCEPTION #10: "I CAN'T GAIN WEIGHT"

There are individuals who often experience a hard time putting on weight. They usually mention "I eat a lot of food, but I stay the same weight" or "I tried eating more food, but it doesn't work". The simple solution is to eat more. You must be in a caloric surplus over time in order to gain weight, which means you must eat or drink more calories than the amount your body burns each day. Your body requires a certain amount of calories just to function and it needs more as you increase physical activity. You must consistently eat higher than this amount of calories each day over the course of weeks or months in order to see a significant difference in your physique. It is true that some people have a harder time gaining weight than others, but these individuals just have to find the right balance of calories that will work for them. The same way your body tells you that you're hungry when you're in a calorie deficit is the same way it will tell you you're full when in a surplus of calories. When most people are full they tend to eat less, which can cause them to not be in a caloric surplus. That is why it can be challenging for some individuals to put on weight if they do not know how many calories they are consuming. It is your responsibility to consume the amount of calories required for you to gain weight whether or not your body tells you if you're full. Though it can be a challenge, knowing what foods are calorie-dense can help you consume more calories without you feeling so full.

MISCONCEPTION #11: 6 MEALS A DAY

You often hear that eating 5-6 small meals throughout the day boosts your metabolism causing you to burn fat. The idea of consuming smaller meals more frequently has an insignificant effect on increasing your metabolism. The main factor that determines the outcome of fat loss or gaining weight is the total calories you consume. If you have 6 meals a day consisting of 500 calories each, that is a total of 3,000 calories. If you have 3 meals a day consisting of 1,000 calories each, then you reach the same total of 3,000 calories. As shown, by eating 3 or 6 meals in a day, you will achieve the same results. Dividing your total daily calories into more meals does not easily change your metabolic rate. Your body takes days or weeks to change its composition, so prioritizing the amount of meals in one day makes minimal difference in burning fat or building muscle. Minor factors such as meal timing is also insignificant toward the development of your physique if you do not have your daily total calories aligned with your fitness goal. An individual should know the total amount of fat, protein, and carbs they need to consume before worrying about how frequent they should eat. Eat whenever you feel hungry as long as you meet your macronutrient goals at the end of the day.

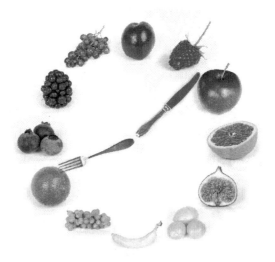

MISCONCEPTION #12: EATING AT NIGHT

When trying to burn fat, many people dread the thought of eating food at night. Though your body is asleep at night, it still uses calories to function and repair cells. You can observe that you weigh less when you wake up compared to the night before due to your body's use of calories. As long as you're in a caloric deficit where you burn more calories than the amount you consume, you will lose weight no matter what time of day you choose to eat. There are diets such as intermittent fasting which proves that you can efficiently lose fat while consuming the bulk of your daily food intake at night as long as the required calories are met. Consuming most of your carbs during the day can be beneficial for having more energy, but this is a preference of the individual and will have no direct effects on burning fat or building muscle.

MISCONCEPTION #13: EATING FAT MAKES YOU FAT

If you are not consuming more calories than your body needs, then eating a high amount of fat will not cause you to gain fat. The main factor that determines whether you gain weight is the balance of calories going into your body and the calories that are burned. With the Ketogenic diet, you can consume a combination of a high fat, low carb, and high protein while still burning fat. On the other hand, it is possible for an individual to consume a low amount of fat while in a caloric surplus, yet cause their body to store the extra calories as fat. One gram of fat is equal to 9 calories while one gram of carbohydrates or protein equals 4 calories. As you can see, fat has more than double the calories per gram than the other two macronutrients. So when you are told to limit your fat intake, it is not because it is bad for you, but because fat is very calorie-dense. There is no set amount of fat that an individual should consume. The key is to maintain a balance of fat that keeps you healthy while ensuring progress toward your fitness goal.

MISCONCEPTION #14: WORKING OUT TOO MUCH

Once an individual discovers the many benefits of fitness, they often become eager to exercise more frequently. With proper nutrition, exercise, and recovery you can train as frequent as you desire. Major factors such as workout intensity, volume, recovery, and amount of calories will affect how often an individual should train. Working out too much or "overtraining" is typically when your training begins to negatively affect other aspects of your health. Signs that one may be overtraining are dizziness, extreme fatigue, trouble with vision or reading, and other unusual conditions. These symptoms are often due to overworking your central nervous system. It is important to know when to allow yourself a complete day of rest in order to limit the possibility of overtraining. Overall, train as often as you desire, as long you provide your body with proper nutrition and recovery time to support your workout regime.

MISCONCEPTION #15: CHANGING EXERCISES SO MUSCLES DON'T ADAPT

You may have heard that you must frequently change your exercises so your muscles don't adapt to your workouts. Ironically, you want your muscles to adapt! A sufficient amount of load on the muscle has to be presented in order to challenge it to grow. Over the course of training, the muscle will adapt to the load that it previously used to struggle with. This muscle adaptation is the growth you are looking for and once it takes place, it doesn't mean you have to change your exercises, but rather increase the load you place on the muscle. This progressive overload can be altered by the amount of reps, sets, weight, or rest time. By progressively challenging the muscle's current condition with greater loads, it will continuously adapt by growing over time. Though you don't have to completely change all the exercises in your routine, switching the order of exercises is sometimes enough to prevent the muscles from adapting to a workout. By making some sort of change in your training you can progressively stimulate your muscles to grow.

MISCONCEPTION #16: FEMALES GETTING BULKY FROM WEIGHTS

Some females at the gym are scared of weight training in fear that it will make them look bulky. Women lack the right balance of testosterone and growth hormones to put on muscle mass the way men do. Most women overlook the amount of effort it takes to build the slightest amount of muscle. There are guys who do weight training almost every day and struggle to put on an ounce of muscle, so females shouldn't be afraid of bulking up with the grasp of a dumbbell. Getting bulky from weight training requires years of training and proper nutrition to support such growth. By the time any signs of muscle growth is even noticeable, an individual should know how to alter their training to suit his/her desired physique. Through the use of diet and a proper training program, it is possible to incorporate weight training without putting on a significant amount of muscle mass.

MISCONCEPTION #17: TOO MUCH PROTEIN

Some may question the amount of protein your body can absorb in a specific amount of time. Your body processes the protein you consume based on many factors. One variable that is commonly overlooked is the other macronutrients consumed before and during the consumption of protein. The amount of carbs and fat in the meal will have an effect on how quickly protein is absorbed. The body can take up to 3 days to completely process certain foods, so the idea of how much protein you can absorb in a small time frame is irrelevant if you are not completely fasted. Large amounts of protein are more capable of being absorbed and properly utilized under certain conditions. For example, more protein is needed in a calorie deficit to decrease the risk of losing muscle. It is ideal to have amino acids (protein) flowing in your bloodstream throughout the day, so it can be beneficial to consume protein with each meal.

An individual's genetics and body composition also has an impact on how much protein their body requires for *optimal* growth. This means a large man will not be limited to the same amount of

71

protein as a small woman. The more muscle you have is the more protein your body will require. If you happen to consume more protein than your body needs, then the excess will be converted to glucose and used as energy through the process of gluconeogenesis (when in a calorie deficit or at maintenance). An individual is recommended to consume a moderate amount of protein during a caloric surplus since excess protein can be stored as fat. Overall, your body is able to efficiently utilize mass amounts of protein as long as it fits the macronutrient requirement that supports your fitness goal.

WEIGHING YOURSELF

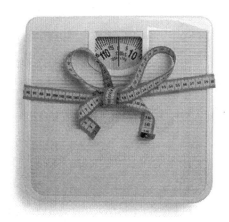

Your bodyweight fluctuates throughout the day, so the scale will display different amounts depending on the time you choose to weigh yourself. Other factors such as how much you eat and physical activity will cause differences in your weight as the day goes by. The most accurate time to check your weight is first thing in the morning after urination. It's beneficial to weigh yourself at least once a week in order to ensure you are making progress towards your goal. It isn't necessary to weigh yourself every day, but doing so will help you get a better understanding of the changes in weight based on your balance of calories.

LOSING WEIGHT TOO FAST

A person can simply lose weight by consuming fewer calories than they burn. This means you can drop several pounds in a few days by hardly eating and tons of exercise. Though this is a sure way to lose weight rapidly, it may not necessarily be the best route to take. Once your body is in a calorie deficit where you burn more calories than you consume, stored fat is used as fuel to compensate for the body's need for energy. But when the calorie deficit is too large, your body will burn more than just fat for fuel. Protein is used as the body's next source of energy, which can cause a decrease in muscle mass. Losing muscle mass usually affects strength and hinders the appearance of your physique.

The goal of losing weight is to burn as much fat as possible while maintaining muscle mass. With that said, it is very important to pace your weight loss when trying to efficiently burn fat. If you drop your calories too much you risk burning muscle as fuel. Studies have shown that losing more than 2 pounds a week puts you at higher risk for losing muscle. Along with the risk of muscle loss, losing weight too fast has further disadvantages such as low energy, mood swings, metabolic damage, and other undesired conditions. Therefore it is recommended to limit your weight loss to no more than 2 pounds per week. The slower the pace is, the more muscle you will maintain.

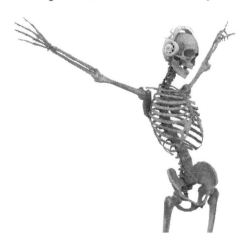

"Patience is bitter, but its fruit is sweet" ~ **Aristole**

BODY ADAPTATIONS

The more you listen to your body is the better you can understand how it responds to what you do. Your body's number one priority is to keep you alive, and therefore has the ability to adapt to the conditions you put it through. The human body aims to maintain homeostasis, meaning it always wants to remain balanced. As your body may often resist changes, it can be challenging to adjust the composition of your physique. An example of homeostasis is displayed while trying to lose weight. When you consume fewer calories than your body needs, it will tell you that you're hungry in hopes that you eat more food. If these signals go unanswered, then the body uses stored fat for the calories it needs. By consuming more calories than your body needs, it responds by telling you that you're full. Ignoring these signals to stop eating will cause your body to store the extra calories as fat. As you can see your body always finds a way to adapt to the conditions it goes through.

The occurrence of body adaptations is also observed in the amount of water you consume. In some cases an individual will drastically increase their water intake during a short period of time and often end up making frequent trips to the bathroom. Eventually your body learns how to utilize this amount of water instead of excreting the abundance. Therefore, it is sometimes best to gradually introduce new conditions to your body and allow it to adapt over time. The human body is a smart and complex system, so understanding how the body responds to what you do, can allow you to better pursue your fitness goal.

"We cannot solve our problems with the same thinking we used when we created them" ~ **Albert Einstein**

HOW CAN I ACHIEVE FASTER RESULTS?

Once you get into the habit of working out, you may be anxious to see the results of the hard work you've put in. The initial thought of achieving faster results is to train harder. Though this will help to a certain degree, it is only a fraction of the formula to reaching your goal. Whether you want to burn fat or build muscle, it is always best to set up a nutrition plan to achieve your goal. Making sure that your plan is accurately set up to reach your goal and actually sticking to it each day is the fastest way to see results. Some goals will take weeks or months to achieve, but by not wasting any days of working towards your goal is the most significant aspect of seeing progress. If you give your nutrition half of your attention, then it can take twice as long to notice the results. Some unbelievable 90-day transformations have come from people who were dedicated to devoting every day towards their goal. If you just kind of want it, instead of 90 days it might take you 180 days or longer, it's up to you.

Making sure your training program is set up to produce the results you desire can be a deciding factor in the progression of your results. Analyze everything you're doing to achieve your goal and figure out what areas you can improve on. Most people are more focused on the training aspect of fitness and hardly pay attention to their nutrition. The more days you dedicate towards improving your training and sticking to your nutrition plan is the faster your results will come.

"Never give up on a dream just because of the time it will take to achieve it. The time will pass anyway" ~ **Earl Nightingale**

WHAT IS THE BEST DIET?

With so many diets out there, it can be confusing to know which one works the best. Popular ones range from Paleo, Atkins, Vegan, Fruitarian, Ketogenic, gluten-free and other mainstream diets. So which one is the best? The best diet is the one that you can consistently stick to the most. All of these diets have one goal in common, which is a method of burning fat. Various diets incorporate restrictions such as emphasizing low carbs, high fat, whole foods, fruits and other regulated guidelines. Whichever diet you choose, it's important to remember that the basic rule of a general diet is to be in a calorie deficit so that you can burn fat. Most people try different diets and restrict all kinds of food but never consistently stay in calorie deficit, which defeats the purpose of being on a diet.

Tracking your macros is a way of knowing exactly how much you are putting into your body, leaving out any room for guessing if you're in a calorie deficit or not. Knowing your macros can help you stick to whichever diet you choose. One diet for example may require you to stay away from bread. This may work for the simple fact that if you ate a lot of bread before and suddenly stopped, then you've lowered your calories, which can cause you to be in a calorie deficit. It wasn't that eating bread was stopping you from losing weight, but because your overall calories weren't low enough. Eliminating certain foods from your diet can help you drop calories to lose weight, or you can keep track of your calories and enjoy all kinds of food within moderation. You shouldn't have to be bored with what you eat so make sure your diet is made up of the foods you enjoy. By following a sustainable diet, you are more likely to maintain healthy habits after you've achieved your goal.

REFEEDS VS. CHEAT DAY

When dieting for some time, people often develop the urge to binge on foods they wish they could have more of. Cheat days sometimes lead to eating more than you're supposed to, which can delay progress towards your goal. Refeeds are commonly known as a controlled cheat day. Having a refeed tends to reduce the urge to binge and relieve the stress of long-term dieting. During a refeed, an individual consumes their maintenance level of calories (or more), which can allow them to eat more food without gaining fat. It is typical to see an increase in weight after a refeed, but it should return back to normal 1-2 days after continuing to diet. The strategy of a refeed is to increase your consumption of carbs for the day while keeping your fat and protein the same. It is beneficial to have a refeed when you experience a consistent decrease in training performance, extreme low levels of energy, or simply as a reward for being consistent with your goal. Incorporating a refeed every week or two during a long-term diet can help avoid any plateaus while trying to burn fat.

ACHIEVING YOUR GOAL WITHOUT TRACKING CALORIES

As simple as anyone can make tracking calories sound, there will always be individuals who still dread the thought of tracking the food they eat. It is possible to achieve a great physique without knowing the amount of calories you consume, but the results can be less *optimal* in terms of time, accuracy, weight-control, stress, body composition, and several other aspects. Though the goal of this section is to inform you on how to avoid tracking calories, it would be extremely useful to keep track of your calories or macronutrients for 1-2 days so you have an idea of how much you consume on a normal day. From this point on, you can adjust the amount you eat and drink based on that amount. A plate-proportion rule can be followed where half of your plate is filled with some sort of lean protein, a quarter filled with starchy carbs, and the last quarter consisting of any type of vegetables. Whenever bulking or cutting, you should always consume at least your bodyweight in grams of protein each day to allow your muscles to recover efficiently.

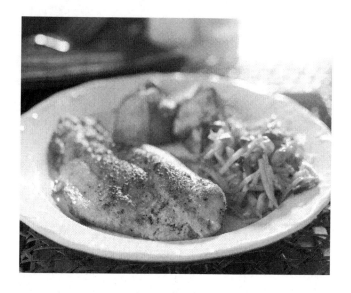

The most important aspect of achieving your goal without tracking calories is to check your bodyweight each week to make sure you're making progress. If you notice that your weight is not moving in the direction you want it to, then you will have to adjust the amount of food in your meals. If you are trying to burn fat, then decrease the carb portion of your meals or limit the amount of fat that you consume. After a few days of staying consistent with your new portions, continue to check your bodyweight throughout the week for any signs of progression. Consuming more vegetables and less starchy carbs can help lower your calories. It's beneficial to only drink beverages that do not contain calories such as water, coffee, tea, and other zero-calorie drinks.

Individuals looking to gain weight should mainly be concerned with consuming more food than their maintenance level of calories. Eating more food than your body needs each day may be challenging for some people. Overtime your body will tell you that you are not hungry, but the key is to keep eating so that you allow your body to gain weight. If you notice that your weight is not increasing each week, then add more starchy carbs to your meals until you see some progression. The downside to not knowing how many calories you consume is that you may gain more fat than muscle if you consistently eat too much. It is also important to remember that in order for the increase in bodyweight to come from muscle growth, some sort of training must be done. Though achieving your goal without knowing your caloric intake is less than *optimal*, these guidelines will help direct you toward your goal.

RESOURCES TO MAXIMIZE YOUR FITNESS POTENTIAL

Information on improving your fitness lifestyle floods the internet each day. There are tons of people who have already achieved their fitness goal and frequently share their thoughts and experiences for the purpose of helping others. It is always beneficial to seek advice that can save you time and energy. Google is an excellent resource to find information on anything, better yet perfect to discover tips on fitness. Youtube is one of the best tools to learn about exercises, proper form, example workouts, recipes, and many other aspects that can help improve your fitness experience. Write down any questions you have about anything you don't fully understand and simply search it next time you're at your computer. It is useful to seek information from multiple resources to make sure the advice you encounter is legit. Instagram is also a great resource for images of great physiques that can help inspire and motivate you to stick to your goals. Use the internet to your advantage and take the initiative to find answers to the things you don't know. The following 'Youtube' channels and websites that have helped me along my fitness journey:

- **PumpChasers -** Outspoken Youtuber with great advice on workouts and meals. Shares his honest opinion on various fitness topics that is sure to entertain.

- **SimplyShredded.com -** High quality content on training, nutrition and personal interviews with the top fitness athletes in the world of aesthetics.

- **Scott Herman Fitness -** Offers detailed advice on how to perform exercises correctly along with footage of example workouts.

- **Christian Guzman Fitness -** Ambitious Youtuber with his own gym and fitness apparel brand "Alphalete", whom vlogs his daily workouts, meals, and business ventures.

- **Nikki Blackketter -** Intriguing Youtuber who vlogs her daily workouts, meals, and life as a fitness enthusiast.

- **Brandon Carter -** Uploads daily videos of quick and simple workouts to do at home with a ton of motivational content for self-development

- **Michael Kory Fitness -** Uploads quick and easy healthy recipes along with frequent workout footage.

- **Athlean-X -** Analyzes the science in building an athletic physique. Critiques individual exercises and offers alternative methods of training.

- **Rob Riches -** Professional bodybuilder who gives professional advice and tips on how to structure your nutrition and training.

- **The Online Coach -** Uploads daily videos of his life as a dedicated gym-owner along with workouts and personal advice on fitness.

- **Twin Muscle Workout -** Twin brothers who share their entertaining opinions on various aspects of fitness.

- **Bodybuilding.com -** The most popular website for information on anything in relation to building muscle or burning fat.

- **Ulisses World -** Professional bodybuilder with great advice and tips on training.

- **Fit Media Channel -** Quality Youtube channel with an inside look at aesthetic bodybuilding and its popular athletes and models.

HELPFUL TIPS

CUTTING

- Drinking coffee can help suppress your appetite
- Don't start your diet too late. Allow a few weeks for your body to make changes.
- Spicy seasonings are shown to help you eat less
- Don't keep foods in the house that can stray you away from your diet
- Keep track of your bodyweight as much as possible
- Chewing sweet gum can help fight sweet cravings
- Adding fresh lemon juice in your water can help you drink more
- Try to stay busy. This will take your focus off of food.
- Eat more vegetables to help you stay full on lower calories
- Limit the amount of times you eat out
- Fit your favorite food into your macros once a week
- Consume protein during the day to avoid going over your carb intake.
- Drink a cup of water before starting each meal

BULKING

- Eat calorie-dense foods
- Stay hydrated. With increased training, more water is needed
- Focus on eating more carbs
- Consume enough vegetables.
- Carry a snack when you're on the go
- Limit cardio
- Focus on training lagging muscle groups
- Check your body weight each week to ensure progress
- Frequently increase the work-load of your training to ensure muscle growth

TRAINING

- Always have a game plan before starting your workout
- Short rest periods cut down on total training time
- Make your workout a priority, not an option
- Learn the proper form before trying an exercise
- Minimize the use of momentum
- Save intense cardio for after weight-lifting or a separate day
- Always try to do better than you did last workout
- Have a music playlist to help you stay focused
- Record the amount of sets, reps and weight for each exercise to ensure progress.

SUMMARY

With many aspects of fitness, there are always improvements that can be made to your nutrition and training. The fundamentals and benefits of nutrition have shown to be applicable to any daily lifestyle. Hopefully it is now understood that there is no such thing as a clean or dirty food, but better viewed as a healthy or unhealthy diet that will direct the progression of your goal. Making a decision to cut, bulk, or maintain weight is the basic foundation for controlling the composition of your body. These caloric states determine whether you burn fat, build muscle, or simply remain the same weight.

The body is extremely smart and will adapt to any way that allows it to function efficiently. By understanding the science of your body, you can make smarter decisions to support the progress of your fitness goal. Your workouts will become more efficient and effective by following the essential training methods and tips provided. In a basic sense, muscles grow with sufficient training, proper nutrition, and enough recovery. It is a cycle that has to be consistently repeated in order to see significant results, making rest and hydration a key role in achieving your fitness goal.

The simple truth of how to burn fat while avoiding the downfalls of common dieting will benefit anyone looking to tone their physique. With many nutritional lifestyles, any diet you choose to follow should include the foods you enjoy eating. It is essential to coordinate your nutrition with your goals while allowing consistency to determine your results. Think of your body as a checklist of daily requirements which include specific amounts of macronutrients, micronutrients, water, and exercise. The more you are able to consistently fulfill all the requirements on your list each day, is the faster your results will come. Understanding the relationship between what you consume and your body's daily allowance, serves you more control, flexibility, and confidence while pursuing your fitness goal. This guide serves as the basic science behind *optimal* nutrition and training that will ultimately lead you to your best physique.

KEEPING IT REAL (PARTING MESSAGE)

There are many people who want to acquire their best physique, but only a few are willing to put in the work that is required. You can read this book a thousand times and study every topic on fitness, but until you take action you will never obtain the results you desire. Many people work hard toward their fitness goals year after year, but still haven't made the progress they expected. Even though it's good to work hard, it is more important to work smart. This book serves as an informative guide with a sincere purpose of helping you make the difference.

Imagine your goal physique and ask yourself, what is stopping you from achieving it. Are the excuses you come up with really worth you not having it? Maybe you just don't want it bad enough, and that's okay. There is someone in this world that has five times as many excuses as you, yet still chooses to do what it takes to go after their fitness goal. Think of those infomercials you see on TV with people who lose tons of weight in 90 days and end up with a toned, muscular physique. You may often think those advertisements are fake and even if they aren't, it would take way longer than 90 days to achieve those kinds of results. Most of the time, these commercials are legit. If you present the same 90-day weight loss program to an average person, they may follow it one day and slack off another day. So instead of 90 days it would take that person 180 days to reach their goal. The only difference is that the people in the infomercials wanted to achieve their goal so bad, they did not waste any days of working towards it. They used their motivation and drive to put in the work necessary to acquire their physique. As cliché as it may sound, this is a true example of the work you put in is the work you get out.

There are people who work out all the time in order to better their physique, yet make little to no progress toward their goal. This is most likely because their nutrition doesn't support the goal they are trying to achieve. Think about trying to grow a plant. You have to place a seed in some soil, expose it to the sun, add a specific amount of water and wait for it to grow. Imagine your body as the seed, exercise as the sun, and calories as the water you need to achieve your goal.

Some individuals provide their body with enough exercise (sun), yet drench their body with too much or too little calories (water) which causes their body (seed) to not develop into the physique they want. You are in always in control of what happens to your body by the choices you make. If you want quicker results, exercise with intensity and be more accurate with your nutrition on a consistent basis. As simple as it sounds, the average person struggles to get it done because their excuses eventually outweigh their motivation for achieving their own goal. Define yourself as being better than average, and go beyond what the average person does.

To pursue and accomplish a goal gives you the confidence to do anything you say you will. Through fitness, you are able to push yourself to become a better individual while directly obtaining the reward for your consistency and hard work. Achieving your fitness goal is a challenge, which is why you don't see everyone walking around with perfect bodies. Without challenges an individual will never grow, so avoid being too comfortable where you are. The human body wants to stay idle and does not want to change unless you force it to. Your mind controls your body, so having the right mindset will allow you to get through any challenges you face. When it comes to pursing any personal goals, the only thing stopping you from achieving it is yourself.

"Knowing is not enough; we must apply. Willing is not enough; we must do"
~ Jonathon Wolfgang von Goethe

ONLINE FITNESS COACHING

It can be challenging to make that first step towards achieving your fitness goal. You may have the motivation to pursue your goal but may not know where to start or may know where to start but lack the motivation to get you through. Whatever the reason is, having a coach to assist you through every aspect of achieving the physique and healthy lifestyle you want is always a great option to consider. With the guidance of your personal nutrition and/or training, it minimizes any guessing out of the process and ensures that you are efficiently pursuing the physique you want. All you do is follow a plan and stay motivated. Here are a few detailed ways that having a coach is beneficial towards reaching your fitness goal:

- **Goals** - Whether you want to lose fat, build muscle, or do both, a plan will be tailored towards your specific goal. Macros and/or meal plan is assigned based on the individual's body type and level of physical activity.

- **Motivation** - While pursuing any goal having the motivation and drive to carry you through is important. Getting bored or off track is least likely to happen with a coach who keeps you motivated and focused throughout the program.

- **Lifestyle & Schedule** - Everyone has unique eating habits and individual schedules that can conflict with their goal. Instead of adjusting your lifestyle to your diet, your diet will be structured around your lifestyle and what is most convenient for you to follow. No matter what traditional foods you like to eat, a coach can choose proportions that will keep you moving towards your goal.

- **Optimal Macros** – With customized macros you maximize the amount of calories you are able to consume while staying on pace to achieve your fitness goal.

- **Accountability** - Checking in with a coach to discuss your progress and how you feel throughout the week will help you stay disciplined towards your goal. If there are any "slip-ups" during your diet a coach will help you get back on track.

- **Personal Advice** - Sincere opinions on food or training is given to help clear up any confusion. Coaches can share personal experiences and offer food alternatives to maintain progression.

- **Timing** - Having a coach ensures that you meet your goal within reasonable deadlines which can include weddings, vacations, or any specific dates. Instead of guessing and hoping your diet works, a coach will help you achieve your goal without wasting any time.

- **Enlightenment** - In addition to your fitness plan, you are also educated about your personal nutrition along the way. This can help you avoid going back to old habits after achieving your goal. Having a coach will help you to transition into a healthy lifestyle that you can maintain and enjoy.

CONTACT INFO

Website: kgfitphysique.com
Email: Kamerongeorge922@gmail.com
Instagram: @KG_FitPhysique

"Nothing will work, unless you do" ~ Maya Angelou

GLOSSARY

Calorie - a unit measure of energy

Caloric Deficit - the state of burning more calories than you consume; a cut

Caloric Surplus - the state of consuming more calories than you burn; a bulk

Caloric Maintenance - the state of consuming the same amount of calories as you burn

Carb - the body's main source of energy

CNS - central nervous system; consists of the brain and spinal cord

Fat - the body's secondary source of energy; controls hormones and helps transport cells

Macronutrient - carb, fat, and protein; large nutrients that contain calories

Metabolism - the process of your body converting what you consume into useable energy

Micronutrient - vitamins and minerals; tiny nutrients that aide functions in the body

Mineral - natural occurring inorganic solid that helps your body develop and stay healthy

Lean Mass - anything in your body that isn't fat; bones, muscle, organs, skin, blood

Optimal - the best or most favorable; most efficient

Protein - supports growth, maintenance, and repair of tissue in the body including muscle

Vitamin - an organic compound that is essential for cell function, growth, and development

Refeed - method of consuming more calories for a period of time during a long-term diet

Sodium - a mineral used to control blood pressure and volume; aides the function of muscles and nerves

Sugar - a simple carbohydrate; different forms include glucose, fructose, and sucrose

Volume - reps x weights x sets; representation of total work done in a workout

BIBLIOGRAPHY

[1] *Learning about calories.* Available from: <http://kidshealth.org/kid/stay_healthy/food/calorie.html>. [December 2014].

[2] Leyva, John, CSCS, CPT, *Whey protein: benefits, risks, & top picks.* Available from: <http://www.builtlean.com/2012/03/16/whey-protein>. [10 June 2013].

[3] Haas, Ryan, *When do muscles grow after working out.* Available from: <http://www.livestrong.com/article/406021-when-do-muscles-grow-after-working-out-with-weights>. [13 March 2014].

[4] Jay, *A list of the best weight training exercises for each muscle group.* Available from: <http://www.aworkoutroutine.com/list-of-exercises-for-each-muscle-group/>. [14 January 2015].

[5] Mayo Clinic Staff, *Metabolism and weight loss: How you burn calories.* Available from: <http://www.mayoclinic.org/healthy-living/weight-loss/in-depth/metabolism/art-20046508>. [19 September 2014].

Made in the USA
Charleston, SC
21 October 2015